Dr. Cass Ingram

M000203846

The Cause *For* Cancer Revealed

...the vaccination connection

KNOWLEDGE HOUSE PUBLISHERS
Buffalo Grove, Illinois

Printed in the United States of America

First Edition

ISBN: 1-931078-17-3

Disclaimer: This book is not intended as a substitute for medical diagnosis or treatment. Anyone who has a serious disease should consult a physician before initiating any change in treatment or before beginning any new treatment.

To order this or additional Knowledge House books call
1-800-243-5242. or 1-847-473-4700

For book information visit:
www.knowledgehousepublishers.com

For product information visit:
www.oreganol.com

Contents

Dedication

To little Mustafa, who is in heaven, where he can no longer be tyrannized—where he is safe from the dirty hands of devious man. To all other 'Mustafas', who have been irreparably harmed by the greed of humankind.

Introduction

There is hope for cancer. This is because it is largely a man-made disease. If the true causes can be determined, then it makes sense that it could be reversed.

Cancer should not be feared. It should be attacked or treated with the proper approach. Chemotherapy and surgery are not the answers, nor is radiation. Rather than cures these are sources of income, that is for doctors and manufacturers, not cures.

That there is a cancer industry which suppresses competition is well known. This industry is based upon corruption arising from the chemical/drug cartel. Of note, a number of the most harsh medicines, for instance, the chemotherapeutic agents, are based upon chemicals formerly used in warfare.

People are poisoned unnecessarily. This is because there are natural cures for this disease.

The chemicals are used because they are a means to maintain the profitability of the chemical-industrial cartel. Here, regarding cancer there is no firm proof that chemotherapy improves life span. The fact is due to this therapy people suddenly die.

There are a number of natural substances which are effective in reversing this disease. How can a supposed cure also kill? Many such medicines have a vast scientific basis. Certainly, such medicines could do no harm. What's more, radical changes in diet drastically aid in the fight against cancer.

None of these medicines or approaches is routinely available. Yet, this is not due to a lack of effectiveness—there are numerous alternative and natural medicines which are proven effective. Rather, it is due to the autocratic actions of the medical/drug cartel, which attempts to crush natural medicine. In fact, during the 1920s through 1930s, when in the United States natural medicine was in vogue, this cartel effectively eliminated it.

What follows is one approach and cure the cartel cannot destroy. This is because the approach in this book is, in fact, the approach of much of the cancer industry. Here, the cure operates in a manner similar to the drugs, except that it is safe and natural. It is a kind of natural chemotherapy. Now the difference is evident: it is safe versus caustic, harmless versus harmful, cause-and-effect versus treating merely symptoms. What's more, in virtually all instances the natural medicines are more effective than the chemicals and are even more curative than surgical procedures. What's more, while they eradicate the cancers they fail to harm the patient. This is the very oath upon which medicine is based: that of Hippocrates, that is above all do no harm. In modern medicine this oath has been completely ignored.

In North America there is an epidemic beyond all comprehension. This epidemic is destroying peoples' health. Most people are unaware of it. This is because the agents responsible operate by stealth. They are insidious perpetrators, which gradually and systematically destroy the immune system. They take control of the entire body, converting it to serve their own objectives. Rapidly, they consume the cells, even causing cell death. These germs are found in virtually all Westerners. The germs are government-issue. They are unnatural. They are artificial, man-made freaks. They are animal viruses, which have invaded the human body. These animal viruses are found in the majority of Westerners. What's more, rather than natural or 'wild' they were created, as well as disseminated, by scientists, who self-righteously claim the ability to cure. This is t virus 40 (SV40) and its associated man-made gerī germs are perhaps the main cause of cancer, the number two killer of Western peoples. Thus, in its arrogance modern science has created a global epidemic.

The name simian implies a natural source: apes. This is precisely the case. However, this is an altered virus, a freak of nature—a hybrid, part human and part ape. It is a laboratory aberration, specifically altered, supposedly to create an immunizing agent—a vaccine—against disease. However, this is an engineered virus, systematically manipulated by scientists. So, while it is monkey in origin, incredibly, even for monkeys it is an aberration. Thus, simian virus 40, commonly known as SV40, which now infects the majority of Westerners is a man-made derivative of the original wild monkey virus. It is the cause of the most widespread and devastating epidemic in the entire history of humankind: cancer.

What a statement it is: that the cause of cancer has been discovered. Yet, this discovery cannot be credited to any of the major institutions: the American Cancer Society, the NIH, NCI, the CDC, or similar organizations. It is not the finding of major medical institutions, for instance, the Mayo Clinic, the Cleveland Clinic, or MD Anderson, although such organizations largely confirm it. Rather, it is the premise of this book, fully supported by the scientific literature.

This is far from a novel discovery. The scientific literature itself reveals its truth. Cancerous tumors are riddled with bizarre viruses, which are foreign to the human body, These viruses aggressively invade it, causing unpredictable damage. These are largely simian viruses—that is viruses from various apes and monkeys—although SV40 appears to predominate.

These viruses don't merely invade the tumors: they cause them. Michelle Carbone, M.D., Ph.D., the primary SV40 investigator, has categorically shown that this germ creates cancers. After being injected with SV40 animals which are cancer-free routinely develop the disease. In virtually all cases test animals develop cancerous tumors, an unheard of statistic. Yet, this is far from a mere statistic, rather, it is an undeniable fact: that SV40 is perhaps the most potent, as well as pervasive, cause of cancer known. What's more, it is a man-made factor, the result of vaccines and other potions given primarily to Westerners. However, a similar vaccine was also given to people in the Third World, particularly Africa. Here too cancers never before known are occurring. Thus, this disease is largely a human creation.

There are other causes for this disease. However, none are as pervasive or traceable as SV40. Other causes have a sound basis, that is scientifically. For instance, the role of toxic chemicals is well established, although, often, it is difficult to prove. Food additives and various processed foods are correlated. A high intake of refined sugar increases the risks for breast, ovarian, bone, and bowel cancer. Nitrated meats heighten the vulnerability to esophageal, bowel, bladder, and stomach cancer. Regular alcohol consumption may cause stomach, liver, ovarian, and breast cancer. Alcohol is also a major cause of mouth and throat cancer. Cancers of the head, neck, throat, and lungs are directly tied to smoking. Pancreatic cancer is correlated with high coffee intake. Margarine consumption significantly increases the risks for all cancers, particularly cancers of the lungs, liver, bowel, and breast.

Yet, even though the role of such factors is fully established absolute proof is elusive. Not so with SV40. The proof is in the tissues: directly under the pathologist's microscope. There is nothing to reproduce, study, or investigate. No prolonged clinical trials must be performed. The evidence is glaringly obvious and beyond reproach. The virus is directly where it would be expected:

within the nuclear material of the tumor cells. Here, it achieves the predictable: it directs the tumor's growth, in fact, causes it.

There is little need to search further. This is the primary cause of the cancer epidemic, which is afflicting the human race and, particularly, which is afflicting North Americans.

SV40: origins

The source of this pandemic is easy to trace. It is the introduction of the highly acclaimed oral and injectable polio vaccines. Few people realize that these vaccines were contaminated, that is with a wide variety of germs. The primary source of these germs was monkey secretions. These secretions were the consequence of the method of creating the vaccine. The vaccine was grown in monkey organ tissue, specifically the cells of monkey kidneys and testes. This includes monkey blood and serum.

Millions of people were contaminated with monkey virus-tainted vaccines. The fact is anyone who received the oral or injectable polio vaccine, as well the vaccine in sugar-syrup, is contaminated. Thus, all such millions are at risk for the development of cancer.

The brunt of the damage was done in North America, where mass vaccination of the population was enforced. Most of the contaminated vaccine was distributed in the United States. The most severely contaminated lots were administered in the states of Iowa, Illinois, Wisconsin, Minnesota, Idaho, Utah, Washington State, Oregon, New York, Maryland, Connecticut, Rhode Island, and Vermont. This is also where the greatest number of adverse events were reported. Idaho and Utah were perhaps the most severely hit, so much so that the head of the Idaho department of health halted the vaccination program. Few Americans are aware of such details: that a state commissioner, so overwhelmed by the acute toxic reactions, canceled a federal program. Was the federal government doing anything other than practicing medicine without a license? Was it recommending anything except medical advice without training, without full knowledge of the consequences? This was a debacle beyond all others. It must not practice medicine. Only competent medical authorities must do so. This was not the case with the polio vaccination program.

This unprecedented and uncalled for action created great harm. The individual might feel anger, certainly frustration—surely pain—at the thought of having been wrongfully harmed. There is frustration and fear. There is confusion. How could such a deadly germ gain entrance to the bodies of hundreds of millions of Westerners—a germ utterly foreign to them? It is a germ from another part of the world, never natural to their bodies. Yet, it infects them, harms them, and, ultimately, kills them. The fact is there is no doubt about it: simian virus 40—the monkey virus originating from imported monkeys—is methodically killing Americans as well as other people. This is merely what must be expected from such a bizarre unnatural contaminant, a venereal virus of wild monkeys. Even famous Americans, for instance, Jackie Kennedy, who likely died of SV40-induced lymphoma, are its victims.

Contrary to popular belief rather than African in source this was an Asian monkey from the Indian subcontinent. Wild monkeys were captured by the villagers and held in cages. Ultimately, they were boxed and shipped via airliners to the United States. Here, the monkeys were kept in farms until they were needed for research. Ultimately, they were sacrificed and their tissues were used to grow the vaccine virus. Monkey tissues are still being used in drug manufacture.

To reiterate there is no doubt that this virus kills. There is no question that it causes cancer, in other words, it creates tumors. It creates novel cancers that were previously unknown. This means that it is a direct cause of human disease and that because of it an untold number of people have been victimized. In other words, these are cancers which would have otherwise failed to develop. These are the consequences of the wrongful practice of medicine upon the public by its own government, without careful medical scrutiny. What's more, this medicine was promoted and endorsed by people who were not physicians and who are not trained in clinical medicine.

How could it be that this could happen in the civilized world? How could anyone do this to people? The people place their trust in the system. The government, they believe, would never harm them. The government is supposed to represent them. Supposedly, the people elected the representatives to serve their interests. It would seem unconscionable that such representatives would violate the needs of the people. Surely, they would only have their interests at heart. Surely, there could be no malice, no intent to cause harm, no purposeful neglect. What's more, certainly, regarding the government it would fail to profit at the expense of the people. The fact is anyone who believes this is naive.

In the United States people believe that the government would never purposely harm them. They believe that it could never intentionally poison its citizens. It was John Lear, in his book, *Recombinant DNA: the Untold Story*, who offered an opposing perspective. That the government would in serving its own interests purposely cause harm to its citizens seems unfathomable. However, that is precisely what happened. Says Lear, essentially;

> 'Profits were placed above human safety, in fact, human rights. The decision was made to protect the pride of the government at the people's expense. A known carcinogen of the most profound degree was purposely disseminated. This is despite the fact that it was proven to be a cancer-causing agent. It was known to destroy human cells. It was an undeniable

contaminant. This was SV40. Yet, it was given to the people regardless. This is indisputable. It is also vile.'

The consequences have been dire: the destruction of lives, premature deaths, a kind of political murder. Yet, no one has been held accountable. No systematic review has been performed. The fact that disease, as well as deaths, have been caused by government policies is beyond dispute.

How could it be: an entire nation, in fact, multiple nations, have been infected with a freakish cancer-causing germ, as well as multiple unknown germs, all by government mandate. Surely, this is a tyranny beyond comprehension. Surely, this is the work of madmen. Rather, it is the work of the devil.

Yet, it should be no surprise that the government would be in the drug-selling business. Since its inception it has earned income on drugs: for instance, tobacco and alcohol taxes. The fact is the government is involved financially in every depraved and destructive influence: prescription drugs, dangerous vaccines, munitions, biological agents, nuclear fuels, nuclear bombs, tobacco, alcohol, gambling, perhaps the opium trade.

To understand the role of SV40 and similar infectious agents it is first necessary to understand the nature of such organisms. It was Wendell Stanley, winner of the Nobel Prize in chemistry for his viral research, who said that viruses are "one of the great riddles of biology." This means that scientists barely understand them. He confirms the long-held notion that outside the body, unlike bacteria, viruses aren't truly alive. They only thrive after invading living beings. In a most fascinating introduction he writes in his book *Viruses and the Nature of Life:*

> *An inactive virus can be seen only with an electron microscope, and then only after it has been "killed (that is fixed with a chemical stain or neutralized by chemicals)." A virus in action cannot be seen at all.*

Furthermore, the moment a virus becomes really interesting, the moment it enters a living cell, it ceases to be a virus (that is it becomes a part of the cell). What is a virus, then? About the only definition that all scientists will accept is: Something. . . . infectious and extremely small, which has the ability to cause disease in almost all living things, and which can reproduce only within living cells.

Obviously, scientists are unsure of what they are dealing with. They know that in cells viruses are an abnormal finding and that, in fact, they disrupt them. Few organisms are so capable of disrupting the integrity of the cells. Viruses are the most aggressive in this regard. In many cases there is seemingly no defense against them. This reveals the danger of manipulating nature—the danger of creating medicines from viruses, that is vaccines. Scientists are unsure what they are dealing with and, yet, they are making medicines from altered germs? This is unconscionable. With viruses, dead or alive, it is the danger of exposing the body to the unknown. The fact is vaccines are perhaps the most poorly tested, that is experimental, of all medicines. What's more, an unknowing population is the guinea pig.

To become alive viruses need living beings, that is a host. This means that they are a kind of parasite. Without them, as Stanley notes, they are as if a "rock": completely inert. Yet, they may become alive at any moment—all they need is a vulnerable cell to infect. What's more, during any such infection they may fail to remain in their original state, rather, they may mutate into totally different creatures, elements never before known—combinations of the old virus and the being it now infects. It rapidly converts itself into a unique being based upon its host.

This is the kind of bizarre machine of synthesis that a virus is—there is nothing else like it in nature. It fully adapts itself to its host, becoming a part of it. Yet, while doing so it damages it. What's more, if circumstances are right, it will kill it.

This is what happened in 1918, when a new virus developed within humans. This virus developed in soldiers from the First World War, who upon returning home or traveling the world, spread it amongst humankind. These soldiers were heavily vaccinated. This is no coincidence regarding the spread of this disease and the soldiers' conditions.

This was the most sudden and extreme epidemic ever to strike the human race—and it originated from the vaccinated. Here, globally, some 80 million people were killed. Rather than an act of nature the fact is the 1918 pandemic was an act of man. Thus, can the injection of viruses into living beings ever be deemed safe?

It is not the people who fail to get vaccinated who are of concern. Rather, it is the vaccinated who will create the next pandemic. They will become breweries for new germs, which will strike human beings suddenly—germs for which they will have no immunity. These are germs fully created by the hands of man, killers which could destroy the human race.

This is already occurring. The hybrids are brewing, and they are seeking vulnerable hosts. Anyone could be the victim, that is without adequate protection. Thus, it is only a matter of time before the massive epidemic strikes. If so, it will be the vaccine industry which is primarily responsible. In other words, in the spread of disease the vaccine will be the culprit. It will be portrayed as if it is an inevitable consequence. Yet, just like in 1918, when inoculated soldiers spread the killer flu, vaccines will again start an epidemic.

After inoculation vaccinated individuals shed germs for up to two months, perhaps longer. Thus, if a global epidemic develops, vaccines must be considered as the most likely source.

Stanley reminds us that of all infections which strike human beings, half are viral. Thus, if a person is sick, especially during the winter, it must be presumed as viral. He then further notes that there is no medical cure for such infections. Yet, there are natural cures that are effective, which this book will demonstrate. Medicine is unable to "conquer" it: however, there are natural medicines—the production of almighty God—which can.

Stanley stresses that viruses are not fully understood. What is known is that they are parasites. How they parasitize cells has never been determined. Incredibly, they are the only known entities that must infect other cells to reproduce. Says Stanley:

> Once inside the cell...it acts as if it were a part of the cell's own complement of chromosomes, and it succeeds in tricking the cell into producing new viruses...the virus becomes an espionage agent capable of extracting from the cell information which the cell otherwise would have kept secret...

In other words, it robs the cell of its secret code for survival and uses it to advance its own agenda: raw survival at any cost.

Viruses are deliberate in their actions: they know exactly what they are doing. Their goal is survival at any cost, even the cost of the host, that is its death. They are among the hardiest of all organisms known, many of which are billions of years old. Thus, viruses are well adapted to attack—even overwhelm—living beings, because they have the most sophisticated, as well as ancient, genetic capabilities possible.

An extremely small error in the reproduction of the virus, as might occur through genetic engineering or vaccine production, could be devastating. Stanley notes that such an error could prove "fatal for millions of human beings." This is the danger of genetic manipulations, as well as vaccine-related production, in the laboratory. Inevitably, such a process is hazardous, that is there is no way to control the outcome of such manipulations. The process easily goes awry and the opposite of what is intended may develop, that is an aggressive killer instead of a cure. The fact is such man-made "errors" will be the source of the next pandemic, the next killer, which will cause the deaths of uncountable humans. Thus, rather than an act of God it will be a man-made event.

It takes only a slight change, a few molecules disrupted, to create a global killer. A single virus has 5 million atoms. If three or so of these are altered, this could make the difference between "a mild virus and a killer..." This is what happened in 1918. It could happen again: at any time.

Viruses are bizarre. They are not really alive, nor are they totally dead. A piece of sand, a bit of rock, a piece of decaying wood: these are all dead, and there is no question of the status. A virus is different. On its own, isolated, it appears dead. However, here too it is bizarre. It appears microscopically like a crystal. It has geometrically perfect shapes. Much like a crystal of, for instance, quartz, viruses exist, plus when gathered together, they form into organized structures, appearing as crystals. Yet, these crystal forming agents can infect living beings. How odd. No one can explain it. They are as if extraterrestrial beings—aberrations from the outer universe. How else could they be explained?

A virus is essentially nuclear material, a genetic crystallization. It is coated for its protection by protein. Once entering the body the the viral coat opens and the invasive material is released. This can spell doomsday for the cells. This genetic material thrives in the vital genetic materials of cells. Here, it blends itself with the living, becoming with it as if one. This is the greatest danger of viruses, to stealthily become a part of an organism. This is why viruses are such an insidious threat. It is also why they are the most worrisome cause of cancer known.

How they infect us

Viruses are invisible. This may shock people. Surely, they can be seen by scientists. Surely, scientists know more about them than this. There must be a mistake. Scientists know well what are viruses, and they can deal with them scientifically. In fact, this is not true. Scientists are unable to see the vast majority of infective viruses, and more correctly they are unable to visualize them while they are infecting tissue, and they are unable to fully understand their operations. In other words, they don't know what they are dealing with. All that scientists can do is speculate. They can see them in an inactive, dead state: fixed on a dead background: but not in a vital, living state. Thus, scientists fail to understand these creatures. This is why modern science has failed to find a cure for even a single viral disease. If medical people, as well as scientists, fail to understand it, surely they could never develop a cure.

Viruses can only achieve a single result: cell damage and death. They may harm a body, severely damage it, or fully destroy it. Thus, the viruses must be destroyed before they destroy the organism. This is the only way to cure viral diseases. It is not to supposedly prevent them with inoculations which, in fact, increase the risks for viral diseases. To introduce a deadly concoction into the tissues: this is a kind of criminal act. No one is helped by such injections: they only create harm. Public protection if any is nil.

It is certain that vaccines cause disease. Thus, as a result of such medicines innocent people are routinely harmed. Entire diseases are largely due to the toxic consequences of vaccinations: autism, attention deficit, fibromyalgia, chronic fatigue syndrome, polymyositis, pericarditis (inflammation of the heart sac), Alzheimer's disease, Parkinson's disease, lymphoma, juvenile diabetes, multiple sclerosis, and various cancers. Is this anything other than professional tyranny of the greatest degree? They are the direct cause of the murderous 1918 epidemic. Yet, despite such known consequences the medical profession righteously imposes such injections upon the people, acclaiming their value. Is there any other possible explanation for this degree of trauma, death, and despair? Vaccinations are directly tied to cancer, in fact, they outright cause it. Thus, how could such medicines be beneficial?

Viruses infect cells, causing vast physiological and structural damage. Says Stanley about the consequences of such infections, "The cells are almost always damaged or destroyed...and when enough cells are affected, we see the result as a symptom..." In other words, all that a human realizes is vague distress, that is various symptoms of unknown cause. He/she has no idea that the tissues are being destroyed. The virus infects and kills insidiously. Usually, no one is aware of the process.

What a bizarre being is the virus. A single 'organism' can kill a person. Yet, microscopically it appears almost inert, like a divinely ordained computer chip. It has no features which make it appear alive. It looks like a gigantic molecule, fully foreign to any known tissue, plant or animal. The fact is it appears as if a microscopic space module. Even more astounding is what happens if billions of viruses are together: they form into a tightly bound and symmetrical crystal: truly incredible. Yet, this geometrical configuration is transitory. When viruses enter living tissue, all changes. No one has ever observed the transition, but it is well known to be true: the virus becomes unraveled, and then it takes action. Once inside the cell it only performs one job: to duplicate itself. This it does by taking charge of the genetic operations. In essence the virus becomes a part of the cell: a frightening prospect.

Obviously, the purpose of the virus is to duplicate itself. However, in the process it often causes rather extreme damage: cell toxicity, cell death, and, ultimately, the death of its host. Stanley again notes that "What the viruses do is to attack... individual living cells and kill them...and when enough of the cells are killed, the animal itself dies." So dangerous are many viruses, he notes, that they need not infect the entire body to do their damage, for instance, in the case of polio: "the viruses may attack only a few cells in the brain stem, but this is quite enough to kill." Unless the virus is killed it will continue to infect and destroy critical cells, with disease or even death being the ultimate result. For the organism to survive the cell death must be halted, and the only way to do so is to kill the viruses. This is the purpose of the immune system. The purpose of the virus is to evade the immune system. The cell has its own virtually insurmountable defense, that is via the cell wall, which blocks viral invasion. However, if the cell is diseased, if there is a defect in the cell wall, the virus may readily enter. Viruses infect the organism one cell at a time.

According to Stanley here is a graphic representation of how this occurs. First the virus approaches the cells, where it sets into motion its invasive process. It becomes attached to the cell, penetrating it. "For several hours after the virus penetrates the cell, we see no changes whatever, although there are profound submicroscopic changes occurring in the structure of the virus...(then) in the center of the cell (is the first change). The multiplying virus particles are first seen within the cytoplasm of the cell, which undergoes degenerative changes. New viruses are gradually released, and finally the cell disintegrates, scattering the remaining virus particles. This process of viral penetration, the multiplication of the virus and its release followed by the death of the cell, is repeated over and over. Each cell releases hundreds, even thousands, of virus particles to infect the surrounding cells. After the cycle has been repeated many times, we have a sizable area of dead cells..."

This method of invasion and killing is typical of the polio, hepatitis, and influenza viruses. Yet, this process, Stanley notes, is only one way viruses cause harm. There is another technique used by still other viruses. This is where the virus is a methodical, systematic killer: the cause of various chronic vague diseases. Here, cell death may occur, but it is in a less obvious way, the gradual decline of health, where the viruses essentially take over the function of human cells, slowly depleting them of all their powers. These are the types of viruses associated with chronic fatigue syndrome and fibromyalgia.

There is yet another type of virus, which is even more ominous: the tumor viruses. These viruses multiply more slowly within the cells than the cell-killing types. Instead of destroying the cells they "cause them to multiply" in an abnormal way. Here, it is crucial to realize that the cell is naturally inhibited for such growth. The fact is it contains specific genes which prevent it. The gene has become inactivated—the virus has taken over that part of the genetic code. This is why the virus must be killed. The fact is by killing it all cancer cell growth is halted. This will allow the immune system to eradicate the cancer.

The role of viruses in the creation of tumors is immense. This is why the role of stealth pathogens, which are vaccine in source, must be investigated. While they may not be the cause of all tumors it was Harry Rubin writing in Dr. Stanley's book who made it clear that viruses do, without any other factor, cause tumor growth, that there can be no tumor, and, then, after infection by a virus, tumor growth occurs. What's more, if the virus is allowed to infect the organism unchecked, the organism dies. Rubin notes that there is no medical cure for such viruses but that if the virus could be killed, the disease process would end. He raises the hope for a chemical cure, which would destroy the virus without harming the cell.

Such a chemical, rather, biological, cure has been found. Rather than man-made it is the chemistry arising from nature. What's more, it is completely safe for use by all peoples. This is the powers of wild spice extracts. Such extracts contain potent antiviral compounds such as carvacrol, thymol, cuminaldehyde, eugenol, polyphenols, and terpenes. It is also through the powers of plant flavonoids, particularly those found in wild fruit. Extracts of such fruit are potent antiviral agents, which offer the benefits of killing a wide range of germs, while increasing cellular defenses.

In 1961 this is what Rubin called for. Then, medicine relied only on chemicals, which damage the cell. The idea of natural substances which strengthen the cells' defenses against viruses, as well as perhaps destroy them, was unknown. Scientists had no confidence in the idea of natural cures. This was the chemists' domain—only man-made chemicals could be expected to cure. This is a philosophy which is still maintained, that is by the medical authorities. Yet, it is now known that such thinking was short-sighted, in fact, destructive. This is because there are innumerable cures in nature and many such cures are even more powerful than standard medicines. The fact is modern medicines originated from nature. The original medicines, aspirin, digitalis, liver extract, high blood pressure drugs, cortisone, etc., all were from nature. The fact is God made all chemicals. When human beings corrupt them, disease, in fact, sudden death, results. With truly natural substances, there is great safety plus, as will be demonstrated throughout this book, the efficacy is far greater and safer. What's more, there is an additional compelling fact: in some instances, the natural substances work more effectively than even the most powerful drugs, while failing to cause serious harm.

The virus is a destructive agent and then another destructive agent is used to further affect the individual. Instead of tearing it down with further toxins why not work with the principle that the natural God-given substances build the body, cell by cell? Through the use of the appropriate natural medicines this is precisely what this book will achieve.

Chapter One
The Monkey Factor

Simian virus 40 is a natural inhabitant of monkeys. It is never inherently a human germ. Then, how did it become a resident in the bodies of over a hundred million North Americans? Incredibly, it was planted there.

The science behind this vaccine was sloppy. The fact is there was no science. In other words, there was no proof that the vaccine was safe as well as effective. It was merely produced in an uncontrolled way and "tested" on humans. The proponents never fully considered the potential harm it would cause.

There were two types of polio vaccines, injectable and oral. The injectable may be regarded as a kind of serum from the flesh and blood of monkeys. The oral type was in the form of a sugar cube, which was soaked in the secretions. There were no independent trials on humans to be certain that this serum was effective. Nor were there any trials with the sugar-cube 'vaccine', that is to ensure safety and efficacy. Nor were there any careful studies to ensure that the oral polio vaccine was safe for babies and children. The fact is this was one vast experiment, with human beings as the guinea pigs.

Sure, medical journals tout vaccines as safe as well as effective. Medical historians claim that because of vaccines diseases have been eradicated—the plagues of humanity, polio, diphtheria, whooping cough, smallpox, cholera, and more. Yet, was it truly vaccines which were responsible? Were these the sole, even primary, factor? Or, were there other factors which were more readily responsible, for instance, the flush toilet, garbage removal, germ-free drinking water, and proper disposal of sewage waste?

There are many examples of disease due to infections, which are clearly related to a lack of sanitation. Diseases which occur as a result of poor sanitation include cholera, typhoid fever, yellow fever, diphtheria, polio, and smallpox. In a sanitation-based society such diseases are rare. In virtually all cases vaccines were introduced during the era of a steep decline in such diseases. Surely, the elimination of cholera has no connection with vaccinations: there were no vaccines for this disease. The same is true of typhoid fever. The latter diseases only occur when there is a breakdown in sanitation. Yet, for instance, with typhoid fever medical authorities, who dispensed vaccines, claim victory over the disease. This is despite the fact that the incidence of this disease steeply declined after the introduction of proper sanitation.

So, the great change in the United States, as well as the rest of the Western world, was the introduction of sanitation. There was another massive change: the mass availability, as well as transport, of healthy foods, particularly fruit and vegetables. Refrigeration prevented food rotting and, therefore, food-borne diseases. Chlorination prevented water-borne epidemics. The introduction of a more varied and nutritious diet prevented physiological collapse and weakened immunity. Thus, the resistance against disease was greatly bolstered.

People in Western society greatly benefitted: their health noticeably improved and, what's more, their vulnerability to epidemic infections was greatly diminished. Farm animals and outhouses were no longer urban. There was running water virtually everywhere. Dirt roads next to homes became virtually unknown. Garbage pickup was mandated. Nests for tens of millions of flies and mosquitoes were eliminated. For the first time in modern history people lived virtually under complete protection, that is the safety and security offered by public sanitation. This was the cause for the massive decline in communicable diseases, not vaccinations.

There is no doubt, that, historically, the diseases for which vaccines are given were killers. Yet, is there any proof that the decline of such diseases is exclusively or even primarily due to vaccinations? It is well established that due to sanitation the former killer diseases were largely halted. Obviously, the elimination of public sewage pits, running sewage near homes, or outflows into public streams would eradicate the dangerous substances and halt disease. Now, the flies and vermin which transmit the diseases of sanitation are eliminated. This is what happened with polio, where it was proven that the majority of epidemics were related to sewage contamination. In the United States virtually all polio epidemics occurred in the heat of the summer; there were no epidemics in the winter. Too, cholera and typhoid fever were almost exclusively summer diseases. Is there need for any further proof regarding the connection? The fact is the drastic changes in public health, hygiene, and sanitation were the primary if not exclusive factor behind the decline of such killers, while vaccines played little if any role.

Yet, even though this disease was declining the medical profession persisted. "To save humankind," it was proclaimed, "a vaccine is necessary." The only way to grow the vaccine virus was in monkeys. So, an extraordinary effort was made to import them. The monkey tissue was harvested and used to produce the vaccine. Then, the vaccine was either injected or given orally to the masses. The monkey-derived vaccine was contaminated with microbes, easily capable of infecting humans. There were hundreds, perhaps thousands, of such contaminants. At least one of these contaminants was a proven carcinogen. This was SV40, a monkey virus of unknown origin capable of devastating the immune system. What's more, this germ rapidly causes cells to turn cancerous. This infection is a primary cause of today's cancer epidemic, all at the brutal hands of greedy men.

People find this difficult to believe, but the fact is the evidence is compelling. There are truly irrefutable facts. These facts are revealed to help people strengthen their bodies and also combat this infection in order to reduce the risks for cancer. It also to provide an alterative treatment for this frightening disease.

Chapter Two
The Cancer Connection

Vaccines cause cancer. There are a number of reasons for this effect. Vaccines are blood products; they are also tissue products. Thus, they contain germs or at a minimum germ DNA. The germs and their genetic material, that is the DNA and RNA, are major causes of cancer. The genetic material alone has been known to be carcinogenic. This dispels the claim that vaccines based upon supposedly dead cells are harmless. The killing of the cells causes the leakage of genetic material: the DNA itself is infective. Thus, the dead vaccines are equally as dangerous as the live-type. Regarding the injection of pathogenic germs, a key feature of vaccinations, this greatly suppresses the immune system. Even the dead or partial components of germs cause immune disruption. Any microbial component contaminates the body. This is because substances act as a tissue burden which the immune system must deal with. What's more, such injections readily cause cellular damage, particularly against the lymphatic system.

Typically, after multiple injections the number of white blood cells in the body declines. Plus, the white blood cells are greatly stressed, as they must deal with the vaccine-induced toxins and pathogens. What's more, it is well known that germs readily invade human cells. Certain of these germs may overtake the native genetic material. In other words, such germs take control of the cellular operations, including reproduction. The germs then cause cancer growth. They then live in the cancer tissue, from which they feed.

The creation of the cancer is necessary so viruses can fuel their growth. Without the cancer they cannot adequately reproduce. Apparently, they thrive on toxic, diseased tissues. Thus, cancer creates the ideal environment for massive growth. Thus, these germs must constantly strive to create tumors, since tumor cells further their survival, while healthy cells limit them. Healthy cells fight viral growth, while cancer cells 'allow' it. Again, the germs must create cancer to thrive. Thus, if such germs gain control of the tissues, the development of cancer is inevitable. Thus, rather than preventing disease the vaccine purveyors, by injecting human beings with germs, in fact, cause it.

To medical people, even the general public, the concept of vaccines is inviting. It seems so simple, so complete. Merely line up for the shot—get that injection. Get the babies and children vaccinated: now they are protected. Now, all is well. Now, the person can be free of fear. No scary disease, no unpredictable epidemic can strike. The individual is supposedly immunized against killer diseases, which might, unexpectedly, attack or even kill the individual.

Yet, is there any scientific basis for this approach? It would seem so. True, in the Western world decades ago there were health debacles, diseases which could maim, cripple, and kill—diseases which are relatively rare today: polio, tuberculosis, diphtheria, measles, mumps, and pertussis (that is whooping cough). It would appear, then, that the vaccinations have helped. After all, such diseases are rare, at least compared to their pre-vaccination rates. Yet, the purpose of vaccinations is to prevent disease, that is to improve health. It is to create a higher level of public health. Here, vaccines have failed. This is because they have, in fact, caused vast disease. In fact, they have directly caused killer diseases, which are responsible for a higher degree of disability and death than the diseases they supposedly prevented. For instance, brain cancer and lymphoma are caused by vaccine viruses. Then, which is more devastating, these or a mere case of mumps or measles? Which is more frightening, the possibility of contracting polio, which is exceptionally remote—hardly one in a million—or the likelihood of developing a massive lymphatic cancer, the direct result of such inoculations?

According to the prestigious cancer center MD Anderson, some 60% of lymphomas are directly tied to vaccine virus, particularly the notorious simian virus 40. This virus derives from the oral polio vaccine, which was given primarily from the mid-1950s through 1960s. This is proof of its role in cancer generation.

Millions of Westerners have this virus in their bodies. The fact is potentially millions of people have contracted cancer from it. So, if the concept of modern vaccines is true, if it is truly a dependable practice—if it is truly a medical miracle—how could it achieve the opposite of its claim, to, rather than prevent the agony of humankind, in fact, cause it? What's more, what proof exists that vaccines prevent disease, that is that they make people healthier, reducing pain, disability, agony, and death? It would appear that it is the opposite: a cause of cancer and various other diseases, including autism, attention deficit, multiple sclerosis, benign tumors, chronic fatigue syndrome, fibromyalgia, pericarditis, vasculitis, rheumatoid arthritis, lupus, scleroderma, eczema, psoriasis, chronic dermatitis, Crohn's disease, ulcerative colitis, and ankylosing spondylitis to name a few. The fact is there are an uncountable number of diseases connected to these injections.

Again, vaccination supposedly prevents disease. If it causes diseases, in fact, a vast number of them, then, can it be healthy? Can it truly be a "breakthrough?" Is it truly the miracle it is touted to be? Or, is it an outdated treatment, which causes a greater degree of harm than benefit? Of what value is it if it prevents certain diseases, while causing uncountable others? What's more, of what value can it be to any degree if it causes cancer?

This is not to claim that vaccinations have never proven effective. The entire concept originated because it was found to be effective: against certain acute diseases, notably smallpox. It was the Chinese who largely originated it. They found that when regarding smallpox if the dried material from the oozing vesicles was inhaled by a potential victim it prevented the disease.

During the Ottoman Empire Turkish physicians found it effective in acute epidemics. If the vesicles from an infected patient were scratched into the skin of the uninfected, this also prevented the disease. These were crude methods, which caused little if any harm. During that era there were no mass-produced vaccines. There was no vaccine industry, which was profit-driven. There was no attempt to use animals to grow vaccines for the human population. There was no mass vaccination of entire populations. It was merely a method used in desperation during epidemics.

During this era there were few if any options. There was no system of sanitation, as exists today. Drugs or herbal medicines capable of killing viruses were largely unknown. Thus, crude methods of vaccination were a logical application. People were dying. All techniques necessary were applied.

The world is different today. Are vaccines even necessary? Or, do they cause more harm than good? What's more, how can any treatment be regarded as a cure, that is if it causes numerous diseases, which were unknown in the population and which cause such a vast degree of chronic disability that entire lives are destroyed?

There is some evidence that vaccines are of value, especially in acute epidemics. However, once the epidemic becomes fully established they are of little value. Rather, usually, they cause more harm than good. What's more, to give them as a kind of preventive medicine in a hodgepodge manner, as is being done for the tsunami victims, also causes great harm. The only time it can be of value is in the midst of a major outbreak, where injections might save lives. Yet, this is only true of certain diseases. For instance, a recent study published at the NIH (National Institutes of Health) found that the flu vaccine was of no value in protecting the elderly. This evaluation of some 40 years of the vaccine's use showed a universal result: widespread vaccination of the elderly was ineffective. In other words, such vaccinations failed to reduce the number of deaths. Thus, the use of mass vaccination appears to be of limited if any value.

Rarely, vaccinations appear to be effective. Yet, even when they are claimed effective it is difficult to tell if this was coincidence or real. For instance, during the late 1800s in Germany smallpox was relatively common. Cyclical epidemics occurred, resulting in thousands of deaths yearly. Tens of thousands of others were sickened. During that era there were no preventive public institutions, for instance, flush toilets or running water. This greatly contributed to the spread of the disease. There was no garbage pickup; no paved roads. Even so, during the epidemics inoculations were attempted. This is where vaccinations are potentially useful, that is short term.

At best vaccines are a kind of emergency medicine. This is because their purpose is served: the creation of greater good than harm. Mandatory vaccination resulted in a drop in the death rate from some 10,000 yearly to 1,500 yearly. Within 15 years the death rate dropped to zero. However, there were a number of deaths attributed to the vaccination itself as well as outbreaks of other diseases directly tied to vaccinations, including syphilis, leprosy-like disorders, and tuberculosis. Vaccine-induced TB itself caused a number of deaths.

As an emergency procedure vaccinations may find use, that is to reduce the death rate. This is the case only during an uncontrollable outbreak, where vast numbers of the public are exposed and no other treatment option is available. However, they must not be given based upon speculation, that is on the basis that a disease 'might' break out. This is what so-called aid agencies are doing in Africa. In this case the vaccine will cause more harm than good. Rather, if ever, they should be applied to help minimize the spread of a known epidemic. This is the most 'scientific' way to use them. This is the determination of the *New England Journal of Medicine* (2001), when the editors proclaimed mandatory smallpox vaccination as unnecessary, in fact, dangerous.

Even so, with the newer science this use is outdated. This is because there are natural medicines which destroy the very germs which cause such epidemics. This is primarily through the powers of wild spice extracts, particularly the oil of wild oregano (P73) and the oregano, garlic, and onion combination, OregaBiotic.

During that period to a degree vaccinations were given for public benefit; there was little if any profit motive. It was a means to cure or halt disease; there were no financial concerns, no board of directors to appease, no pressure to "create" profits. Today, the vaccine industry is compromised due to the lust for financial gain. Quality control is compromised. There is always a rush to create the proposed seasonal vaccines. Thus, the lust for profit and market share supercedes safety. This has resulted in the public's loss.

Vaccinations should only be given under specific medical indications, where the benefits far exceed the harm. Plus, before they are given they must be proven safe. In other words, the public must not be experimented upon. Otherwise, at least in modern Western society their use should be curtailed. The truth of this statement will be demonstrated throughout this book. This is because it will be thoroughly shown that, today, they cause more harm than good. It will clearly be demonstrated that people are becoming sickened by vaccines, while little if any disease is being prevented.

Yet, there was another difference in that earlier era, where vaccinations showed some benefit: the fact that such vaccines were a kind of crude natural product, though not without side effects, but, still, natural. There was no genetic engineering, no drastic alteration of the natural structure or physiology of the germ, as there is with genetic engineering or other 'modern' techniques. Nor were there any harsh drugs or chemicals added. Today, vaccines are genetically engineered, which greatly heightens their toxicity.

No one knows for certain the long-term consequences of such substances, injected into the human body. Gulf War Syndrome is evidence of the danger where tens of thousands of veterans have developed chronic diseases. These diseases have been attributed to the genetically engineered vaccine. Humans are experimented upon. There is no proof that such engineered vaccines are safe. In other words, no testing has been done to ensure safety or efficacy. It is an experiment upon humankind, and the results are disastrous.

A number of modern vaccines have been genetically engineered, and in virtually all cases they were not tested—the testing is merely the injection into unsuspecting humans. This means that from the point of view of the drug cartel humans are mere guinea pigs. Perhaps this is why modern vaccines are fraught with problems, including the development of frightening diseases, inflammatory disorders, shock, neurological diseases, and even sudden death. This is why such vaccines are among the most potent carcinogens known.

This purpose of this book is to give a factual assessment of the benefits versus risks. There is no attempt to merely bash an industry. Rather, the objective is public safety, that is what is best for the individual. The possibility that properly made vaccines could help minimize an epidemic is real. Yet the plethora of data shows that, long term, the risks are greater than any benefit. The SV40 pandemic has clearly proven that.

How vaccines are manufactured

According to *The Illustrated Family Doctor*, published in the 1920s, the term vaccine means "...preparations containing *disease germs* injected beneath the skin in the treatment or prevention of diseases caused by those germs". From this statement a frightening picture develops. It is of the use of a toxin to 'cure' disease. The authors continue to explain the contents of these vaccines as being either "...living germs...but as a rule...dead germs." The injection, they claim, constitutes a "quantity of liquid containing a certain number of germs (5, 20, or even a billion germs per dose)...so that an accurate dosage can be carried out." Regarding the manufacturing procedure they note, "the germs are grown from secretions or blood..." This confirms that vaccines are blood products.

Blood is the most dangerous of all substances, the cause of fulminant epidemics. Major killers of modern times: AIDS, hepatitis, immune deficiency, mad cow diseases, and numerous others are all blood-borne. The fact is blood is contaminated with untold types of germs. A single milliliter contains thousands, perhaps millions, of species. Plus, there is no guarantee that the supposed sterilization process used in the manufacture of vaccines is effective. Recent evidence indicates that in virtually all vaccine germs survive and if not the actual germs, certainly, germ DNA. The DNA is far from innocuous. Once in the body it can become activated, splicing itself into cells.

Even the older vaccines were problematic. Ida Barnes, M. D., and the editors of the *Household Medical Advisor* note that various systemic diseases, including tuberculosis and some types of syphilis, that is spirochetal infections, can be transmitted through vaccinations. What's more, they may even be contracted through close contact with the vaccinated. Thus, say the editors a monumental effort must be made to ensure that the vaccine 'serum' is "free of contamination," that is that the animal 'lymph' is free of disease. This demonstrates the danger of using animal matter as a medicine.

Surely, in that era the health of animals was superior to the health of today's cattle. What's more, these early authors claim, if truly healthy herds of cattle are used to 'grow' the vaccine, there is little danger of "contaminations."

Even so, the *Advisor* fails to recommend wholesale immunization. Rather, it is to be used for specific cause: to block predictable epidemics. Say the authors regarding the concept of preventive vaccination unless at a time of great danger, "a child should not be vaccinated, that is unless in good health and until it is six to twelve weeks old." In other words, the authors were well aware of the catastrophes caused by immunizing newborns. Such authors take a special precaution against arbitrarily injecting infants, babies, and toddlers due to concern of serious side effects, perhaps fatality. In contrast, in the United States without any monitoring babies are routinely immunized.

Even newborn infants are not exempt. They routinely receive the poorly tested hepatitis B vaccines. Regarding the latter there is no proof of safety, nor is there any proof of need. Incredibly, by the time a child is two or three years old he/she may receive as many as 40 vaccinations, an unmerciful load of toxins and antigens. Yet, the recommendation of the earlier authors is correct. This is proven by the Japanese regulations, where children are never vaccinated until their immune systems are more mature.

In Japan vaccinations begin at two to five years of age. This is because the Japanese are well aware that, immunologically, infants and toddlers respond poorly when overloaded with this therapy. This coincides with a recent Japanese article, Kumagai's work, published in *Pediatric Allergy and Infectious Diseases Society*, that when vaccinated with the flu vaccine, infants did poorly. The investigators determined that the vaccine damaged their immune systems as compared to people who fail to get vaccinated controls. This demonstrates that the Japanese are correct in their approach: babies and infants should not be vaccinated. Their immature immune systems are incapable of withstanding the toxic load, let alone the plethora of additives and chemicals contained in these potions, which are used to preserve and liquefy them.

This is not to deny that vaccines might prove valuable, even for infants, but only if the benefits outweigh the risks, for instance, in the midst of a developing epidemic. Yet, today, there are options far superior to vaccinations, that is the use of nutritional support as well as potent natural medicines. This may, in fact, antiquate the use of any vaccine, that is if such an approach is applied systematically. Again, while temporary immunity may be achieved through such injections—although if the Japanese research is to be believed this is doubtful—the long-term consequences must be considered. Vaccines are produced from blood products. Such products are contaminated. This contamination will result in disease.

Since the early 1900s it has been well known that a variety of pathogenic infections can be introduced through vaccination, even tuberculosis. In fact, as described by Horowitz in a well researched monograph the entire modern (1920s through 1930s) tuberculosis epidemic may have been caused by vaccinations, since the vaccines were derived from the secretions of cattle and TB was endemic in them. Even venereal disease has been attributed to vaccinations, since, obviously, if animals are infected with such germs, these infections are transmitted into the vaccine solution. The fact is if animals harbor infection the final product will be contaminated. Is it even reasonable to suspect that the vaccine industry only uses healthy animals or that they even have the ability to truly determine an animal's health?

Yet, the question regards risk versus benefit. Is the risk of the vaccination—the reactions, toxicity, chronic disease, and sudden death—higher than any protection? In the case of the modern use of vaccines evidence points to significantly greater risk than benefit. Even with the pandemic diseases of the past there is little evidence that vaccines were anything other than a short term treatment, that is to minimize the scope of the epidemic. Even here their effectiveness is questionable. What's more, in many instances, clearly, vaccinations perpetrated the epidemics. This is true of the 1918 killer flu which originated in vaccinated soldiers, as well as the 1958 polio outbreak, which also originated due to inoculations. Thus, the value of vaccinations as preventive medicine is suspect.

Other measures proved far more significant, including sanitation. The introduction of the flush toilet is directly correlated with a decline in the major killers of the time: cholera, typhoid fever, smallpox, and similar infections. Regarding typhoid fever the benefit of vaccination was marginal if any. Surely, the proper elimination of sewage wastes and garbage was far more significant. This is proven by the following chart produced by the United States Office of Surgeon General:

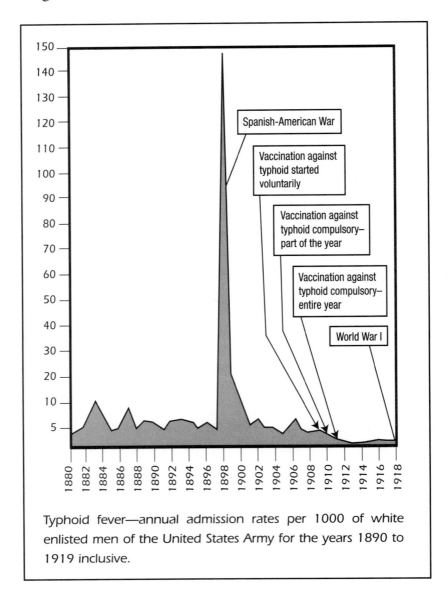

Typhoid fever—annual admission rates per 1000 of white enlisted men of the United States Army for the years 1890 to 1919 inclusive.

Chapter 3
Danger Zone

Vaccines are poisonous. This is far from a radical or biased statement. The fact is they contain known poisons, for instance, mercury, aspartame, and formaldehyde. A poison which is injected is far more toxic than one which is ingested.

Blood and other secretions are contaminated with a wide range of germs. The only way to 'sterilize,' that is render safe, such secretions is to treat them with chemicals. Here, the most noxious possible chemicals are used. Residues of such chemicals are impossible to remove from the treated secretions. Such residues remain in the final product.

Since the beginning of the vaccine industry a wide range of toxins have been used in attempt to render the vaccines safe. This is merely an attempt to reduce the infectivity of the vaccine: to prevent these products from causing acute infections and, potentially, sudden death. This can never be fully achieved. Certain microbes have proven resistant to such chemicals. What's more, the chemicals themselves cause disease. There is another factor which is even more diabolical: genetically engineered, that is altered, germs. Numerous vaccines, including the hepatitis B vaccine, which is routinely given to babies, are produced with this technique.

The use of this method is criminal. It is never based upon science. Rather, it is mere guesswork. As a result, lives are put at risk; catastrophes are created. The entire motive is profit oriented: to create a patented medicine. Genetically engineered vaccines have fared poorly and have proven more toxic than naturally derived ones. Plus, genetic engineering requires the use of even a greater number and degree of chemicals than the typically naturally produced solution. In addition, during genetic engineering toxins are produced by the organism, which may have an exceedingly high potency.

These are far more toxic than any naturally occurring chemicals. This occurred with genetically engineered tryptophan, which was produced by artificially designed bacteria. These bizarre bacteria—man-made freaks—synthesized toxins, which proved highly damaging to human organs. As a result of the toxins produced by this fabricated bacteria, which fully contaminated the tryptophan batches, tens of thousands of people were sickened. This was known as Eosinophillic Myalgic Syndrome, a new disease: all due to genetic engineering. Incredibly, as a result of the ingestion of such a product tens of thousands of people fell seriously ill; some fifty died. This disaster was caused by the federal government, which approved the genetic engineering process. Thus, the introduction of genetic engineering in vaccine manufacturing merely potentiates the toxicity.

Monkey blood, urine, and semen

Simian virus 40 naturally infects monkeys. Here, it causes no known diseases—so it is claimed. It is never a natural inhabitant of humans. Particularly for North Americans other than perhaps zookeepers and exotic pet owners there is no real means to contract this virus. However, now it lives in the vast majority of

Americans as well as a high percentage of Canadians. In England a high percentage of the population also has it. This is also true of many Europeans as well as Russians. In particular, the latter were heavily vaccinated, particularly during the experimental phase. Within such individuals it causes a smoldering infection, which can ultimately lead to cancer. The fact is contamination by the virus has led to a pandemic of proportions which are beyond comprehension.

Monkeys are the natural host for this germ. Unscrupulous scientists had been growing the virus in monkeys in an attempt to create a supposedly useful strain, that is for creating medicines. Researchers used the cells of monkeys, notably from their kidneys, as well as testicles, to grow the viruses. Essentially, a viral brew was created: viruses require animal tissue, in fact, animal blood and secretions, to grow. The polio viruses were added to the solution, which consisted of mashed monkey kidneys and testes, and allowed to grow. Obviously, such a solution also contained a variety of secretions, including monkey blood, urine, seminal fluid, and sperm. This high nutrient-protein solution greatly encouraged viral growth: untold trillions of viruses were grown. The purpose was for the manufacture of vaccines. The resulting solution was treated with chemicals and then turned into an inoculation: the modern polio vaccine. Then, the vaccine was distributed throughout North America, particularly the United States. Tens of millions of Americans, primarily during the mid-1950s through 1960s, were inoculated with this contaminated solution. Such people were never informed that the source of the vaccine was infected monkey cells or that it was grown on monkey blood or tissues. To do so would have caused a public outcry—people would have refused to take it.

Informing the public was a conflict of interest. This was an enormous business. Yet, rather than medical authorities it was an industrial operation mandated by the government, not by medical authorities. The fact is there was little if any medical basis for such a vaccine. What's more, it was never fully tested for safety or effectiveness.

The process for making the vaccine was as follows: monkey kidney cells, that is the cells of an excretory organ, were used as the growth medium: the viruses were added to the cell culture. The cells were colonized by these germs, where they reproduced. The cells were eventually processed and the contents extracted. The resulting solution was used to create the vaccine: essentially, a monkey blood derivative swarming with viruses.

The mass vaccination program initiated by the government had no science behind it: no firm medical basis. There was no solid proof that the program was either effective or safe. Only later, some five years after the program was initiated, was the degree of danger discovered.

In 1955 the program was begun. The contaminant was discovered in 1960. Much of the damage had already been done. Monkey virus was seeded into virtually every American family. The virus readily shed, that is through the stools, urine, and oral secretions as well as through the sexual fluids. It could even, so the government determined, be spread orally.

No one knows for certain what was done in those labs: how the virus was grown and/or manipulated. How were the cells cultured? What chemicals were used in the process? Were the viruses altered or manipulated? Was their genetic structure disrupted? Did the viruses convert into a mutated form, after being treated with antibiotics and solvents? Was a super-germ created, a Super SV40? Studies in the wild indicate this. When humans who are regularly exposed to wild monkeys are checked, the fact is there is evidence of SV40 exposure. However, what is ominously absent is any evidence of tumor causation. What's more, if the wild type is injected into test animals, they develop tumors, but it is not nearly as aggressive in creating cancers as the type found in the polio vaccine. This indicates that the type of SV40 which infects Westerners is a bizarre mutant, a freak created at the hands of man.

When injected into research animals, simian virus causes brain cancer. This alone should cause all authorities to tremble. This means that the government itself is the progenitor of deadly disease. The government, anxious to avoid any discrediting of the public health system, disguised the findings. The fact is it failed to recall the tainted vaccines, even though millions of such doses could have readily been confiscated and destroyed. Instead, knowing full well the danger and scope of the contamination it turned a blind eye. In contrast, the health of millions of Americans was placed at risk. The fact is from 1955 to 1963 nearly 100 million Americans received SV40- contaminated vaccines. This was through primarily the sugar-cube vaccine, that is the oral polio vaccination as well as the polio injection.

Today, the statistics are frightening: some 61% of all new cancer patients are infected with SV40. These are largely people too young to have received the contaminated vaccine. Thus, this virus is transmissible, both sexually and in utero.

SV40 is known technically as a polyoma virus. The suffix "oma" stands for tumor-initiating. Such viruses thrive by creating tumors. This type of virus is a DNA virus and contains a type of structure that allows it to readily insert its DNA into the hosts' cells. This means that regardless of the host it may readily create tumors: this is what it is designed to do.

The ability of this virus to create tumors has been known for over 50 years. Its tumor-producing properties were first reported in 1964 in the *Journal of the American Medical Association*. Yet, in the government offices this was known as early as 1960, some three years before the vaccine was administered.

This virus is particularly likely to invade or damage traumatized tissues as well as inflamed or ulcerated regions. In other words, if there is a weakened or diseased tissue, this is where SV40 is frequently found. Here, it acts as an opportunist, taking over weakened cells and inserting its DNA. It splices itself into the host DNA, overpowering the genetic machinery. It then causes the cell to mutate, so that it can serve its insatiable needs. As described on the Web site BioElectric, "scientists are amazed at how little genetic material these viruses carry in proportion to the damage they can cause."

Another source on the Web is equally compelling. This is the highly credible chronicillnet.org. Here, the writers interviewed the key source—the man who originally discovered the contamination, the government's Dr. Ben Sweet. It was he who first revealed that all batches of the Sabin oral polio vaccine were hopelessly contaminated. His article, the first produced in Western literature warning of the dangers of monkey virus infections, was published as a paper, *The Vacuolating Virus: SV40*. In this article he divulged an ominous concern: that other unknown simian viruses lurk in vaccine solutions. Leveling with the interviewers Sweet's comments were revealing:

> No one really knows if there are any dangers, but no scientist can definitively say there aren't any, that is what's scary...(Regarding SV 40)...It was a frightening discovery, because, back then, it was not possible to detect the virus with the testing procedures we had. It only showed up in the cells of the African Green monkeys—the species being used exclusively by our company. We had no idea of what this virus would do thirty years ago.

Regarding the implications of their findings Sweet continued:

> First, we knew that SV40 had oncogenic (cancer-causing) properties...which was bad news. Secondly,

*we found out that it hybridized with certain DNA virus,
like adeno virus, such that the adeno virus would then
have SV40 genes attached to it. We couldn't clean up
(the double contamination, that is the virus had fixed
itself to another virus: it couldn't be removed)...*

This is a dire finding. It is the establishment of a gruesome fact,
that is that tens of millions of Westerners have been infected
with a vicious agent, which establishes itself permanently
within the body. What's more, this is confirmed by the very
researchers, who, working for the government, did the original
research. The researchers discovered the contamination in a
timely basis. The septic batches could have been pulled, in fact,
destroyed. However, the government chose not to do so and,
instead, placed untold millions of its citizens at risk for the
development of sudden or chronic diseases, which threaten
their lives. This is the legacy of a system—the capitalism of
Western civilization that people throughout the world
seemingly admire—which places business interests above the
needs of the people. Thus, does capitalism mean anything other
than capitalizing upon any opportunity regardless of the
consequences? Does it mean anything other than profiting at
any cost, even the cost of human lives?

Chapter 4
Chaos

Vaccines are a major cause of human harm. The degree of disability they create is beyond comprehension. The fact is modern vaccines have ruined untold millions of lives. There are no human studies which prove that they are safe. Rather, in most instances the human body responds poorly to such injections, which leads to the development of bizarre diseases. Infants or toddlers with weak systems may react violently, resulting in a rapid decline in health, even sudden death. In children with weak immune systems deadly diseases may develop such as rheumatoid arthritis, asthma, seizure disorders, muscular dystrophy, cancer, and diabetes. In teenagers and adults, usually, chronic diseases develop, for instance, eczema, psoriasis, nephritis, chronic fatigue syndrome, fibromyalgia, chronic pain, neurological disorders, and perhaps cancer.

Such diseases may never have developed were it not for the inoculations. Yet, due to fear and perhaps ignorance Westerners continue to abide by the system—the very system which is causing their demise. People continue to maintain that the government, that is the system, would do them no harm. They fail to realize that the government is a business, not merely an altruistic organization.

Vaccines are a major cause of disease, being directly responsible for certain illnesses. These are illnesses which prior to the introduction of modern vaccinations failed to exist. Such illnesses include chronic fatigue syndrome, aplastic anemia, ankylosing spondylitis, lupus, fibromyalgia, polymyositis, polymyalgia rheumatica, scleroderma, and numerous kinds of cancers, particularly lymphoma, bone marrow cancer, and leukemia.

Unless these viruses, that is the various simian viruses which have invaded human cells, are purged, the likelihood of the development of cancer is virtually certain. These are highly aggressive germs, which virtually immediately upon invading the body cause cancer to develop. The body attempts to resist this, but, ultimately, the virus wins.

Such cancer causing viruses would appear to be inborn. These viruses may also create benign tumors, however, their specialty appears to be cancers. This is why since their discovery they have been known as oncogenic viruses, meaning cancer-causing. They are also known as vacuolating, meaning they destroy the insides of the cells, leaving them as empty shells. Apparently, cell death, as well as cancer tissue, helps fuel the virus's growth. Unless the immune system is dramatically bolstered and the virus is diminished or destroyed, cancer will eventually develop.

In humans these viruses serve no productive purpose. Rather, they are deadly. Their existence is for a single purpose: to destroy the human cells and to create cancers. There is no natural defense against them. These are mutants created in the lab. They are aberrations, freaks of laboratory science. They can never be fully controlled or killed by the immune system. A more powerful force must be administered. This is the force of nature, specifically in the form of wild spice extracts. In other words, the viruses must be safely purged from the body: without harming the organism. This is what the wild oregano can achieve. As documented by a plethora of modern research, including studies at Georgetown and Cornell Universities, spice extracts, notably oil of wild oregano, oil of cinnamon, and wild cumin oil, are potent antiseptics. Such extracts exhibit significant antiviral actions. They are even capable of killing animal viruses, including SV40 (note: these are active ingredients of a high potency formula known as OregaBiotic). What's more, spice extracts are general germicides, meaning that they kill a wide range of viruses. Regarding vaccine contamination this is critical, since there are likely numerous other simian viruses simultaneously infecting humans. Thus, a viral purge is required, that is for a satisfactory cure to be achieved. What's more, the spice extracts are capable of purging virtually all pathogens which might be associated with this infection, such as molds, yeasts, and bacteria. These vaccines may also contain highly potent chemicals, known as mycotoxins. Such toxins are capable of damaging the internal organs, including the lymphatic system, immune system, and brain. The fact is spice oils aggressively neutralize such toxins, wild oregano oil being the most powerful.

The infestation by this virus, or, rather, group of viruses, is real. The virus penetrates deep into human tissues, thriving only within cells. In fact, it lives in the cell nucleus. Here, it creates a kind of genetic warfare to fully take control of the cellular functions. Thus, it overtakes the cell's protective code, converting it to a kind of viral hybrid. In other words, the simian virus takes control of the cell, using it for its own purposes. The fact is it is the most efficient parasite. The infection has spread throughout the Western public. Americans are the main victims, followed by Canadians, Britons, Europeans, and Russians.

Lymphoma: a monkey virus disease?

Prior to the era of vaccination in the United States the incidence of lymphoma was low. Only about two per hundred thousand developed it. Since the early 1950s the incidence has climbed dramatically, doubling by about the mid-60s. Over the past thirty years it has mysteriously doubled again, which has mystified investigators. Now the mystery is uncovered. Investigators at MD Anderson confirmed the cause. They studied frozen sections of lymphoma tissue from a variety of patients; in nearly six of ten cases simian viruses were found. The virus fully infected the tumors and, rather, seemed to cause them. This is because it was discovered that it exists on the so-called suppressor cells, the native cells which block cancer growth. This is clear evidence that lymphoma is a monkey virus disease.

William Carlson's article, published in the *San Francisco Chronicle*, March 2002, bravely expounds the connection. According to Carlson:

> Scientists have found traces of a monkey virus that contaminated the polio vaccine in the 1950s in a common form of a highly malignant human cancer that has mysteriously doubled...over the past 30 years. Two studies published...in the British journal Lancet found a link between the virus, called SV40, and non-Hodgkin's lymphomas, a disorder ranked fourth or fifth among cancer deaths in the United States...Results suggest that the virus may play a much wider role in cancer than previously suspected.

Regarding the vaccine he notes:

> The Salk polio vaccine, administered by injection in the United States and worldwide from 1955 through 1963, was grown on minced kidney tissue from rhesus monkeys. At the time the manufacturing process was

*considered safe. But in 1960 it was discovered that large
batches of the vaccine were contaminated with the
simian virus later named SV40. An estimated 90 million
Americans received Salk vaccine injections and as
many as 30 million were exposed to the virus.*

To demonstrate the degree of risk from vaccination he writes:

*SV40 may be involved in a much broader group of
human cancers, playing a...role in nearly half of the
55,000 new cases of non-Hodgkin's lymphoma
diagnosed annually. The cancer, which can be highly
aggressive, has been associated with HIV-positive
patients, and it was through the suppression of the
immune system in these patients that may have had a
connection with the dramatic increase in lymphomas
since 1970 (note: it takes several years for this cancer to
develop—the simian virus was inoculated into humans
primarily from 1955 to 1964, a revealing timeline). The
new studies examined lymphomas from HIV-positive and
-negative patients. Results suggested that both groups
had either about the same level of SV40 DNA fragments,
or that the HIV-negative samples had a greater incidence.
The second group of researchers were at the Fred
Hutchinson Cancer Research Center in Seattle and the
University of Texas Southwestern Medical Center in
Dallas. Remarkably, both groups...using slightly
different detection techniques came up with almost
identical results: SV40 fragments were found in 42
percent of the 154 lymphomas sampled in one study,
while the other found 43 percent in 68 cases.*

Then, he describes a kind of controversy, in fact, a
government conspiracy. The government, says Williams, holds
to the statement that there is "no conclusive proof", that the
vaccine causes any disease. Thus, the government created
disinformation to diffuse public concern, the same process

traditionally used in the former Soviet Union. In contrast, independent investigators claim the connection strong: "Dr. Adi Gazdar of the University of Texas...said...that the "data is very, very solid." He said it had to be more than coincidence that the four types of tumors found in hamsters after injection with SV40—brain, bone, mesothelioma, and lymphomas—are now exactly the same tumor types in humans found with detectable levels of SV40. According to Dr. Gazdar the chances are 10 million to 1 it is a coincidence." Thus, the government claim of "controversy" or "lack of proof" is debunked. Finally, he notes that "U.S. officials have all but ignored the detection of SV40 and that government funding and support for research has been nonexistent.

Gazdar among other scientists makes clear the reason for the government attitude: it is that it is worried about its role in "promoting polio vaccination campaigns." It is also because the initial press on SV40 was that it caused only bizarre or rare tumors. Says Gadzar, "But you can't ignore lymphoma; it's too widespread and too important a cancer. Jackie Kennedy and a lot of other well-known people have died from it."

The making of the devil

It was in the United States where the polio vaccine was popularized. Rather than scientifically based it was largely politically inspired. In culminating the program there were also major business interests. Here, the vaccine was developed and manufactured by private companies. This is in contrast to the Netherlands, where it is made in government-funded labs. The bitter rivalry between the doctors of the original polio vaccines, Salk and Sabin, was a contributory factor to the U.S. catastrophe. This was because there was a rush to market, which compromised safety.

It was a bitter rivalry: two men vying for fame and fortune. The science was poor and was skewed for personal gain. The evidence for human safety was lacking, as was any solid evidence for cure. Yet, the program proceeded, fully funded by taxpayers. The claim is that these vaccines were tested, supposedly offering protection. There is no guaranteed proof of this. However, it was nationally published that during a clinical 'trial' involving thousands of people the Salk vaccine was supposedly some 90% effective, or at least so were the media claims. Sabin's vaccine was touted at nearly 70% effective. There was no independent confirmation for such claims.

In fact, industrial production facilities were built with funds from public donations. This was in advance of any study. The fact is even before the study was done these facilities were ready to operate. Testing was done mainly on Americans. With Salk taking the precedence with a higher supposed cure rate, undeterred, Sabin accelerated his efforts. Another group, Cox and Koprowski, like Sabin, worked on a live-altered vaccine. Both of these groups experimented with their vaccines largely offshore, for instance, in Northern Ireland, the Congo, Latin America, and Russia. By mid-1960 some 15 million Russians are said to have received Sabin's oral vaccine. These men became exceedingly wealthy through multi-million dollar grants.

Sabin rushed his vaccine to attempt to unseat his rival. Neither followed strict scientific protocol. Salk left much of the detail work to mere lab technicians, busying his time in business endeavors. The famous pictures showing Salk holding up tests tubes in a white lab coat are the result of a March of Dimes orchestrated publicity stunt. Thus, incredibly, it is no surprise that the vaccine would be contaminated. The fact is despite full awareness by Salk of the existence of contaminants the vaccine was launched. Yet, it is the Sabin vaccine which was most heavily contaminated. This is because the latter was based upon the giving of live viruses and, thus, every dose—every sugar cube—was teeming with billions of infective organisms.

The government used the media to hype the vaccines. The mandatory program was a success: all of America and much of the Western world followed protocol. Ultimately, the relentless effort of Sabin payed off: his vaccine took precedence, and the injectable Salk vaccine fell out of vogue. Sabin's vaccine offered the benefit, so the government touted, of creating 'passive' immunity. Such terminology, which caused the vaccine to seem innocuous, was part of the propaganda campaign. This is because the vaccine caused active infection of the bowel, which resulted in the excretion of the live but altered virus. This biological freak, it was proposed, would then through the waterways and ultimately through tap water offer immunity to all citizens. Plus, during defecation the virus was shed; this too supposedly disseminated the immunization. There was no proof of this: merely presumption. It was all theory, but it was so thoroughly promoted that it became as if truth. Americans never doubted it. What's more, the school system supported this tyranny, making all such vaccinations mandatory.

Throughout the Western world the Sabin vaccine became readily accepted. By the 1970s most Westernized countries had adopted it, and it became a vast global enterprise, the makers reaping hundreds of millions of dollars in sales. The World Health Organization recommended it for poor countries. This was through a nebulous organization known as the Expanded Program of Immunization. It was even foisted upon countries where polio was essentially unknown. Again, this is despite the fact that there was no proof that the vaccine was safe. The market for the vaccine continued to grow as the authorities pressed the program into more and more countries. Soon, vaccine facilitators were operating in virtually all poor countries, administering their noxious wares without safeguards.

No one considered the potential adverse consequences. It was "right" because the all-knowing WHO, as well as the U. S. Department of Health, mandated it. Now it is known that the polio vaccination may have created untold millions of chronic illnesses, devastating the health of entire populations.

Consider the African continent. Much of the chronic illness which plagues the population developed after mass vaccination. Diseases never before seen—those typical of modern Westerners—now plague the population: chronic fatigue syndrome, fibromyalgia, polymyositis, lupus, juvenile arthritis, diabetes, multiple sclerosis, thyroiditis, Addison's disease, endometriosis, leukemia, lymphoma, brain tumors, arthritis, cancer, and untold other syndromes. Thus, the vaccines caused a genocide. Prior to the vaccinations in such areas no such diseases occurred. This is compelling evidence that the vaccines are a cause of disease, not a preventive. Today, with the mass vaccinations of the victims of the tsunami a further genocide will result. The fact is now people who were relatively free of vaccine-related diseases will develop them in a fulminant fashion and will be dependent upon the medical system for life. The only dilemma is this is an area where support for vaccine injury is nil. Thus, untold thousands will suffer a harm that would have failed to occur had they simply trusted in destiny. UNICEF and similar criminal organizations heavily vaccinate the survivors for essentially non-fatal diseases, and, incredibly, the result will be chronic disorders, even cancer. Do not donate funds to criminal organizations, which without substantiated science or proof of safety enforce the pharmaceutical agenda.

With the introduction of vaccines Third World countries are experiencing epidemics of AIDS and AIDS-like syndromes. No such epidemics were experienced prior. Do not forget: in modern vaccines human cells are used as a growth medium. Such human cells could likely be infected with AIDS or AIDS-like germs. The source of such cells is aborted fetal tissue, and it is well known that the AIDS microbes are transmitted sexually as well as absorbed by fetal tissue. There is no way to fully screen cells for such disease-causing germs. Fetal tissue is inherently infected and, what's more, the degree of infection depends upon the degree of exposure of the parents. Despite testing within fetal tissue bizarre germs, such as syphilitic-like organisms, AIDS-like viruses, cytomegaloviruses, various fungal forms, and, of course, the SV40 and its facsimiles—all can be transmitted, directly into the vaccine solution. Even with chemical treatment, as is demonstrated by the SV40 epidemic, there is no guarantee that such germs will be purged. What's more, certainly, there are other unknown germs which infest fetal tissue, the degree, again, dependent upon the degree of exposure/disease of the parents. Sperm readily transmits infections. So do the female secretions.

Nearly 50% of all North American men have SV40 virus in their sperm. The damage caused by Sabin, as well as Salk, in their reckless pursuit of fame is incomprehensible. What a vile deed it was, and what vast damage was caused to the entire human race. These men have caused a greater degree of human misery than perhaps any other medical men of modern times. This is because the SV40 which they generated is the primary cause of cancer in Western civilization. Thus, Albert E. Sabin and Jonas Salk singlehandedly are responsible for millions of deaths and untold other millions of cases of dire illness, including entire categories of illnesses: mesothelioma, non-Hodgkin's lymphoma, and a rare kind of brain tumor (known as choroid plexus), the latter being exclusively due to the Sabin/Salk vaccines, rather, defilements. Thus, Sabin and Salk earned fame and riches, while causing despair, agony, and death.

SV40 causes other diseases: immune deficiency, AIDS-like syndromes, chronic fatigue syndrome, fibromyalgia, polymyositis, lupus-like syndromes, ankylosing spondylitis, chronic arthritis, scleroderma, multiple sclerosis, myasthenia gravis, benign tumors, particularly of the brain and bone, and chronic lung disease. It is also a major factor in chronic weak immunity: a vague condition, where the individual's immune system is constantly under siege. This may be manifested by a low resistance, low white count, reduced globulin levels, and an overall sluggish ability to fight infections. Sabin clearly stated that he wanted to be known as the modern Pasteur: for him fame was all. This is directly due to the aggressive nature of the SV40 and similar viruses, which invade the immune tissues, damaging and destroying the immune cells. SV40 is capable of attacking all immune cells as well as the cells of the internal organs.

The white blood cells suffer immensely under the pressures from the various simian viruses. These viruses invade such cells, cannibalizing them—consuming their nutrient stores, invading and manipulating their DNA—and, ultimately, destroying them. This is why in terms of blood testing a true pearl of SV40 infection is a low white count. If this is accompanied by a low blood globulin level, as well as, perhaps a low albumin level, the diagnosis of SV40 infection is virtually confirmed.

It seems unfathomable, yet all this agony is due to human corruption. It is the greed and avarice of a few men: power-brokers in the government, haughty medical professionals, greedy businessmen, and self-styled humanitarians, that led to this catastrophe. Sabin himself became a wealthy man. His objective was personal, perhaps financial, never humanitarian. He served the government and the medical/pharmaceutical cartel, not humankind. He sought only fame and wealth and pursued it with recklessness. This has led to the destruction of many lives, the premature deaths of uncountable thousands, the primary victims being Americans.

Perhaps Sabin and Salk truly believed in their approach. Yet, they failed to conduct the proper scientific investigation to ensure that their theories were correct—to be certain that their therapies were safe as well as effective. Yet, since the incidence of polio in the United States was plummeting was there any sound reason to enforce mandatory vaccination? Why treat a disease that is massively declining? Why treat perfectly healthy people for a disease that is such low risk and do so with an invasive therapy of unknown risk?

Sabin and Salk were competitive. The fact is there was a vicious campaign between them for the national contract. Polio was in a steep decline. The flush toilet, sewage processing, chlorinated water, and garbage control had seen to that. This was a stool germ; if fecal contamination was eliminated, its culmination was a matter of time. The likelihood that a supposedly preventive vaccine would add to the cure—a vaccine made from the blood, testicular secretions, and urine products of animals—was nil.

The Salk vaccine was introduced in the mid-1950s, at a time when in the United States there was a 90% decline in cases. Sabin was an aggressive marketer, plus he had a vendetta against his colleague. His vaccine (note the use of the term 'his') displaced Salk's, largely because it was more convenient, being soaked into a sugar-cube. Virtually, the entire civilized world adopted it. In the process this man became a multi-millionaire and world famous. Somehow, quickly, he was awarded a Nobel Prize. This was before there was any proof for his claim, that is his propounding of a cure. In contrast, as a result of his vaccine hundreds of people, mostly fully healthy individuals with no history of paralysis, in fact, developed polio. This is a sickening crime. It is a crime, because public safety was compromised for the sake of business interests. Yet, this was not just any safety issue: this was the heightened risk for enormous misery of humankind: the risk for cancer-causing infections and other infestations that lead to chronic diseases. In what is an unlikely coincidence after the mass polio vaccination program there was a vast increase in chronic diseases, particularly neurological disorders and various previously rare cancers.

Yet, was this the necessary consequence for the cure? The data fails to support such a claim. The Sabin vaccine failed to prevent disease. Statistically, polio was in a decline. If it would have been in an epidemic state and, then, the vaccine was introduced followed by a decline—then it would have been possible to determine its effectiveness. However, there is no possibility to claim it was effective, because of the already rapid decline in the rate of the disease. Thus, any claim for curative potential is specious, in fact, an utter fraud.

Sabin and Salk are far from the sole perpetrators of this *crime*. The March of Dimes must also be held responsible, since they promoted the claim for cure, convincing the gullible public. As a result of the Sabin/Salk vaccine lives were destroyed—people were killed.

How can a cure kill anyone? How can it kill hundreds of people? How can it cause permanent paralysis, nerve destruction, and muscle dissolution? Fatigue, exhaustion, muscle weakness, and muscle atrophy—can a cure cause these? Yet, all such conditions were the direct result of the Sabin/Salk vaccines. What's more, how can entire new cancers, let alone the Western cancer epidemic itself, be synonymous with a cure? It cannot be: it can only be treachery—the cause of disease, rather than the cure. Polio was not cured by the Sabin/Salk vaccines. It was cured by an improvement in infrastructure, by the installation of modern facilities, by improved hygiene, by chlorination of water, and by the elimination of septic wastes. It was the modernization of the Western world which eliminated this disease, not vaccines.

There is a House Subcommittee, which is reviewing claims of negligence by the government. This is in relation to specific human victims, who are suing it. The victims are represented by Stanley Kops, an attorney who says he represents people who were paralyzed, severely wounded, and/or killed by the vaccine, which was in use until 2000. Kops alleges that the manufacturer, Lederle (now owned by Wyeth), as well as the FDA, was negligent. What's more, he claims that they failed to protect American children.

The vaccine, known to be contaminated with animal viruses, was used until 2000, when it was discontinued. Incredibly, suddenly, after nearly four decades of mandating it its sale was prohibited. This is critical, because it is popularly believed that only the early recipients of vaccines were/are at risk: the people who received the admittedly fully contaminated vaccines given from 1953 to 1964. Since then, the government insisted, there was no further contamination. Still, ground animal kidneys are used to grow the virus, particularly from monkeys. This was the source of the original contamination. Yet, it has been righteously maintained that the contamination has been resolved and that only the original recipients of the vaccine, those given the oral polio (sugar-cube) between about 1960 to 1963, as well as those given the shot from 1954 to 1963, are contaminated.

Since then, supposedly, the vaccination was 'safe.' This is because, so the authorities claim, the original source of SV40, rhesus monkeys, are no longer used and, instead, the SV40 virus-free monkeys are the source. The drug company's own internal documents dispute this. Incredibly, according to the documents in Kop's possession it appears that Wyeth-Lederle continued to use rhesus monkeys as a source of cells for growing the vaccine. This would perpetuate the SV40 epidemic, putting children, as well as adults, at risk for aggressive cancers. That the original vaccine, that is the seed used to incubate vaccine manufacture, was tainted is without question. Yet, the issue is: are the vaccine manufacturers continuing to use the original stock? In all likelihood this is the case. Thus, the contamination is impossible to resolve.

Says Kop there is a history of negligence involving Wyeth-Lederle. Wyeth, which now owns Lederle, paid little heed to manufacturing protocol. SV40 screening was often neglected. Different species of monkeys were used, many of which were likely infected. There was no 100% check on these. Besides SV40 there are a variety of other simian viruses, which are highly pathological. Few if any of these were tested for such pathogens. What's more, at Wyeth there is a well known history of contamination, where entire labs have been closed down due to the crisis. Vaccine safety tests, which are required by the government, were not submitted. The regulators failed to investigate this. As a result, contaminated material was shipped and injected into babies and children. As a result, some infants/children became paralyzed. Others died. What's more, he notes, there are now "clear instances of cancer reported in the children...who received this product." Some of the documents he uncovered in his discovery include:

- an original letter from Albert Sabin to Lederle Labs saying that the original seed used to create the 'Sabin' vaccine is not guaranteed to be free of SV40.
- a statement by Wyeth's head of biological control that the unit fails to routinely test monkeys to be sure they are SV40-free.
- company protocols demonstrating that a cell batch used to make vaccines might be accepted, even if SV40 was found.
- an internal memo showing that the monkeys in question, the rhesus species, are, in fact, still used as a source of cell culture. In contrast, Wyeth had previously denied it.
- a 50-year-old or so letter from the pharmaceutical firm Merck & Co. to the U. S. Public Health Service saying that the company would fail to engage in the manufacture of a Sabin-like, oral, vaccine due to the exceedingly high risk of SV40 contamination. The company told the government that it is too difficult to eliminate monkey viruses and that they are virtually undetectable.

Chapter 5
Conspiracy to Kill

Polio is largely a man-made disease due to human excesses. Historically, it is readily determined that this is a disease largely due to poor sanitation. The germ itself is an intestinal virus, which is a normal inhabitant of many humans.

Early research determines the true source of this epidemic. It also determines the corrupt nature of the vaccination program. The following is derived virtually verbatim from a comprehensive survey written in 1956 by M. B. Bayly, a British medical researcher. Some of the terminology has been adapted for the sake of easier reading. This is a highly credible review based upon the actual facts of the time. It is not anti-pharmaceutical propaganda.

According to Bayly in his article, *The Story of the Salk Anti-Poliomyelitis Vaccine,* in 1908 polio was first transmitted to monkeys by two scientists, Landsteiner and Popper. Soon thereafter it was observed that monkeys which survived one attack became resistant to further infection. This suggested the use of serum from human victims who had the disease for the treatment of any victims. A serum derived from recovering children and adults was introduced for this purpose in 1911 and was widely used, being promoted in the press for several years.

However, ultimately, it was abandoned as useless. Then, in 1917 Pettit promoted the use of serum against polio derived from inoculating a horse with monkey nerve tissue which was infected with the virus. He later obtained an antiserum by inoculating a chimpanzee with the same method. However, neither of these serums were effective. Even so, the research continued, with strains of polio being adapted to grow in other animals, including mice and rats. All such germs became mutants, true freaks which never occurred in nature. Then, in 1949 it was discovered that the polio virus grew well in tissue culture.

Microbiologists manipulated such viruses until they developed novel, that is man-made, strains. They believed that they had stumbled upon a cure: potentially 'non-infective' polio strains that could possibly be safely injected into humans. So, during the 1950s investigators created specialized polio strains, a combination of different types. They had no idea what the consequences would be. The purpose was to create a weakened variety that could massively be injected into humans. Thus, this was truly a man-made type of polio—a virus that would only rarely cause the disease. However, could it cause unexpected diseases such as cancer? During that era this was a concern. Yet, no testing was done to ensure against it. However, the polio virus now in hand had its issues. It was a man-made virus, combining cultures grown in various animals, including monkeys and rodents.

No such virus had ever before been introduced into humans. This was truly an experiment, and unwitting humans were the test creatures. Obviously, the long-term consequences were unknown. What was obvious was that in the majority of recipients it failed to cause the sudden disease—full or partial paralysis—so characteristic of true polio. Yet, how could such a reaction be expected in the majority—the fact is this could only be anticipated with the wild type. The vaccine virus was a man-made corruption, so if it did cause disease, it would be an unknown reaction. Incredibly, researchers failed to consider this and only sought comparisons with the naturally occurring type. A report from 1954 clearly documents that this is a man-made virus of multiple animal origin and that mice and monkeys are at least partially the source. This means that at a minimum children are being injected with (or taking orally) a potentially destructive virus, which may cause unknown consequences, even cancer, certainly neurological diseases. The fact is no virus derived from monkeys and/or rodents can be fully safe. This fails to include the issue of unknown contaminants. This issue was, in fact, addressed with a dire warning, even in that era.

It was Dr. James McIntosh, Professor of Pathology at the prestigious London University, who, when addressing the Royal Society of Medicine, said, "Scientifically, it cannot be disputed that from every point of view the injection of a virus *capable of multiplying in the body* (which the Sabin vaccine was capable of doing, even though it was taken orally)...is bad. When multiplication of the virus occurs, then there is no possibility of estimating the dose to which the patient has been subjected. Thus, the effect cannot be controlled, and in susceptible individuals this may lead to *unforeseen results*." Dr. McIntosh proved prophetic, seeing that, today, SV40, which was inoculated into humans from the polio vaccine, is a primary cause of infectious cancer, as well as neurological diseases, such as ALS, Parkinson's disease, muscular dystrophy, and multiple sclerosis. Incredibly, Sabin himself found proof of McIntosh's prediction, when he discovered that as soon as a tiny amount, a mere drop, of supposedly harmless vaccine virus was given to human volunteers, the viruses converted to a highly aggressive form. In other words, they developed into pathogens.

Monkeys in the wild are one thing. However, to capture and bring them to the human world is another. What follows is a rendition of the original 1950s description of how this occurred:

An interesting account of how the Salk vaccine was made appeared in *Time* (March 29, 1954). The story begins with the trapping of rhesus monkeys in large numbers in the north Indian state of Uttar Pradesh. These monkeys were stuffed into cages and carried on shoulder-poles to Lucknow. A train journey of 260 miles took them to New Delhi. A transport plane carried them the 4,000 miles to London Airport. From London another plane transported them an additional 3,000 miles across the Atlantic to New York. They traveled in trucks for a final 700 miles to Okatie Farms in South Carolina. There, these rhesus monkeys from India were caged with other hordes, that is of 'Java' monkeys from the Philippines.

According to *Time*, "It was the University of Pittsburgh's Virus Research Lab where the bulk of the work was done and the vaccine initially produced. Dr. Salk, who pursues his investigations here, has behind him 81 million dimes (some eight million dollars, an enormous sum at the time)...This is part of the three billion dimes (300 million dollars) subscribed by the public to the National Foundation. But in order to vaccinate the million children as proposed in the 1954 tests it was necessary to hand over the manufacture...to five pharmaceutical firms, Parke Davis & Co., in Detroit, Pitman-Moore and Eli Lilly & Co. in Indianapolis, Wyeth, Inc. in Philadelphia, and the Cutter Laboratories in Berkeley, California. For all of them we are told, "the indispensable material is the monkey..."

Just how this was done was never before publicized:

> ...some 50...monkeys will be used in a single morning. Under anesthetic a surgeon removes the kidneys, after which the monkey is killed with an overdose (of anesthetic). Then, the kidneys are cut into tiny pieces and placed in glass bottles with a special nutrient solution devised by Dr. Salk. These bottles are then rocked in a mechanical machine for six days in an

incubator to stimulate the growth of the kidney cells. At this state fluid containing live polio virus is introduced and the bottles again rocked. After about four days the virus has multiplied a thousandfold in the kidney cells and is now chilled in 21 gallon bottles ready for transportation (to the pharmaceutical houses). There, the brew is filtered free for the kidney cells (which might cause nephritis if injected into a human being) and diluted with formaldehyde to kill the virus.

As we have already seen there are three main strains of polio virus, against all of which there is need for protection. Consequently, three tankfuls each containing one type of virus, cultivated and killed in the above manner, are mixed together. After neutralizing the formaldehyde with sodium bisulphite, there is a process to see if the vaccine is safe for injection into human beings. This necessitates inoculations into live monkeys, rabbits, guinea pigs, and mice. These tests are carried out simultaneously, on each batch issued, by Dr. Salk's laboratories and by the National Institute of Health at Bethesda, Maryland. Having passed the final tests the vaccine is distributed...for inoculation into children.

Before this complicated procedure could be devised Dr. Salk and his staff engaged in a long investigation to discover which part of the anatomy of the monkey provided the most useful virus-growth in cells. Like John H. Enders of Harvard they came to the conclusion that this was the kidney, but a leading article in the Lancet (April 18, 1953. p. 777) stated that the testicles, as well as the kidneys, are used as a source of the cells, which form the culture-medium. Monkey tissue is apparently preferred to human tissue, because it has been pointed out, it is more readily available and also because human material might contain the (hepatitis *virus). Despite the known risks from human tissues at least one country, Sweden, continued experimenting with the production of a vaccine derived from virus grown in human fetal material.*

The timing of the vaccine's launch is telling. It was on April 12th, 1955, the tenth anniversary of President Franklin Roosevelt's death, that the Foundation told the world, using all available means of publicity, that the vaccine devised by Salk was "safe, potent, and efficient." This is because it was on this day that the eagerly awaited report on the 1954 tests of the vaccine was issued by Dr. Thomas Francis of Michigan University; it was he who had been entrusted with evaluating the results. At a meeting of 500 doctors and scientists at Ann Arbor, Michigan, Drs. Salk and Francis made such sweeping claims for the vaccine that nearly every American newspaper declared that Dr. Salk had abolished polio, this even before the vaccine had been administered.

Before there were credible reports regarding the effectiveness of the vaccine, six manufacturers had received orders from the Foundation. This was to produce enough vaccine to inoculate 9 million children and pregnant women (therefore, giving Western children, particularly Americans, the very germ which causes cancer). Two hours after the announcement by Drs. Salk and Francis the government licensed the vaccine and released it for distribution to all the states that had agreed to use it. The British newspapers and, particularly, the scientific journals were more guarded. This gives further proof that rather than medical the program was government-based. The cautionary advice by the British was justified by subsequent events, as was the attitude adopted by (the British) Ministry of Health.

Thirteen days later the vaccine was acclaimed by the whole of the American Press and radio as one of the greatest medical discoveries of the centuries. What's more, two days after the

English Minister of Health announced he would go ahead with the manufacture of the vaccine came the first news of disaster. Children vaccinated with one brand of vaccine had developed polio. Then, a few days later additional cases were reported, some of which occurred from yet other brands (that is other drug houses). Then, another unanticipated complication arose. The Denver Medical Officer, Dr. Florio, announced the development of what he termed "satellite polio", that is cases of the disease in the parents or others in close contact with the inoculated children (this failed to account for numerous outbreaks of pseudo-polio such as multiple sclerosis and muscular dystrophy). This occurred, even though, initially, the children had been vaccinated in hospitals, where they remained for a few days and who, even without any major symptoms of polio, still communicated the disease to others. In other words, these vaccinated individuals, free of obvious polio, gave the disease to unwitting contacts. Within a matter of months government offices had confirmed some 150 cases of polio in the vaccinated, with six deaths, and some 150 cases among the close contacts. Thus, rather than a cure the vaccine was a public disaster.

The deaths due to the vaccine could not be taken lightly. Public health officials were appalled by the toll, many of whom called for the cancellation of the program. This represented a greater number of deaths at that time from the vaccine itself than could be expected from the actual epidemic. The American public had been the unwitting victims of a marketing scam, and they were fully unaware of it.

There were a few brave public health officials who took independent action: Utah and Idaho cancelled mandatory vaccination. The officials there saw too many disasters—naturally, there was little polio or various neurological disorders in these regions. The sudden increase in illnesses was obvious and compelling. Here, in the healthy outdoors epidemics were unknown. Almost immediately, public health officials noticed abnormalities—as well as sudden death—and immediately halted the campaign.

This was no minor issue. The deaths and illnesses due to the vaccinations were obvious; the statistics weighed against the vaccinations. Thus, the cure rapidly was revealed as a fraud. No matter; the propaganda machine pressed on, so that the public never truly understood the consequences, in other words in many regions where the vaccine was administered the incidence of polio rose dramatically, as did the incidence of polio-like illnesses such as partial paralysis, Guillain Barré syndrome, and muscular dystrophy. Then, no one made the connection, except those few state and local health authorities, to whom it was obvious that the vaccine was dangerous.

At the time that the vaccination was introduced the American public was relatively healthy. Public sanitation was largely in place, and, so, major outbreaks had become rare. There were no obvious epidemics, particularly in the wealthier regions as well as in the middle class. What outbreaks did occur revolved around the summer and were, obviously, directly related to a lack of proper sanitation. Then, suddenly, after the vaccine was administered Americans fell ill, with many middle and upper class individuals even contracting the full-fledged disease. There were over a hundred cases of complete paralysis. What's more, polio-like illnesses broke out in high numbers, that is in numbers never before seen. There were outbreaks of multiple sclerosis, myasthenia gravis, and muscular dystrophy, all seemingly directly related to the vaccine. Concerned public health officials were appalled. The contamination was so significant that the maker of the worst vaccine, Cutter, was forced by the government to halt production. Yet, regarding the accidental, that is satellite, cases, the situation was far worse.

This is because children were converted into carriers of the disease; their immune systems might handle it, but they might give a potentially fatal infection to vulnerable individuals such as the elderly or a person with a weakened immune system. This is precisely what occurred: the children were turned into human viral bombs, depositing and disseminating their infectious secretions at will. As a result untold thousands, perhaps millions, were incidentally infected. Some died, others were paralyzed, and still others were left with the vulnerability for chronic diseases, including neurological disorders and cancer. This is yet another legacy of the Sabin/Salk vaccine parade, the most poorly conceived public health program in the history of humankind.

As reported in the *Daily Express*, May 16, 1955, a catastrophe developed in Denver, Colorado, where some 1500 children received the contaminated vaccine, that is the type that could cause active polio. Said the investigator at the time, Dr. Florio, when inoculated with a faulty vaccine, children become carriers of the virus. Said the doctor, "We have created a group of carriers...and then there will be another group, and so the cycle will go on. It is very distressing." It was further noted that some of the victims, that is the contacts of the children, will develop the disease in the most severe form, in other words, some will develop permanent paralysis.

The period between the injection and the first signs of paralysis ranged from 5 to 20 days. What's more, in a large proportion of the cases it started in the limb where the injection was given. Another feature of the tragedy was that the number of people who developed polio was far greater than would have otherwise been expected without the vaccinations. In fact, in Idaho according to a statement by Dr. Curl Eklund as written in the *News Chronicle*, May 6, 1955, a chief virologist for the government, polio struck that year only in vaccinated children.

This was in areas where there had been no cases since the preceding autumn. What's more, in 9 of 10 cases the paralysis occurred in the arms where the vaccine had been injected. This led Mr. Peterson, Health Director of the State of Idaho, to call for a halt to the mass inoculation program. According to the *Daily Telegraph*, June 19, 1955, he stated, "We have lost confidence in the Salk vaccine. This outbreak has resulted in 86 cases of the disease, including seven deaths, since the mass immunization program began in April. Mr. Peterson expressed disappointment that scientists and officials had not visited Idaho." He contended: "This was the H. Q. of the biggest outbreak there was. This was the place where they could study the facts." An article in *Time*, May 30, 1955, noted, "In retrospect a good deal of the blame for the vaccine snafu...went to the National Foundation (that is March of Dimes), which, with years of publicity, had built up the danger of polio out of all proportion to its actual incidence and had rushed into vaccinations..with patently insufficient preparation."

For a concise and sober judgement on the catastrophe it would be difficult to better the statement which appeared in the *Medical World News Letter*, June 1955. Under the heading "What We Think" the editor wrote: "There is a useful lesson to be learned from the *sorry story* of the Salk polio vaccine in the U. S. A. It is that a new therapeutic measure of the fundamental importance should not be launched until every possible medical and social implication has been considered."

The March of Dimes itself is essentially a government agency. It served to use the polio crisis for its own designs. Polio was a sympathy card for collecting donations. The funds were largely spent on promotion, advertising, and administration. Little if any was spent on independent science. Thus, rather than an altruistic or scientific effort the entire project from the funding to the design—to the decision to employ Sabin and Salk—was a government project. The name was coined by actor Eddie Cantor as a play on the newsreel, *The March of Time*. The idea was to raise money from schoolchildren and others, who would contribute dimes to the cause. This is why President Roosevelt is on the United States dime. This was a public relations gimmick. The fact is there was no scientific basis for this program. Polio was on a massive decline. Perhaps there was an attempt to capitalize upon this sickness, before it was exterminated.

Polio is a fecal germ. It thrives in wastes. America was rapidly becoming 'sanitized.' The era of untreated sewage waste and stagnant filth was rapidly ending. So was polio. Summer outbreaks were becoming more rare. The medical profession had no basis for recommending a mass vaccination campaign and did not support such an action. The recommendation came from the government, or, rather, business interests. There was no sound medical basis for it, nor was there any medical consensus to support such vaccinations. Incredibly, children, with the countless dimes collected, paid for their own harm, perhaps demise.

The pharmaceutical houses have long dealt with blood, and vaccines are blood products. This is a fast means of making money, while holding a monopoly. When the war ended, so did the blood business. This is because war injuries must be treated, and this requires various blood products, all of which are produced by the pharmaceutical houses.

This has not always been the case. Prior to the 1900s there was no "blood industry." At the beginning of the 20th century the pharmaceutical industry was made up of mainly regional companies. Only a few such companies were national. There were thousands of small makers, many of whom made food-like and/or herbal extracts.

Many such companies made high quality natural products. Doctors throughout the country touted these medicines for their curative, as well as safe, actions. However, during the 1930s the medical profession waged a vast war against natural medicines, even though many of these medicines had been proven effective. If the medical monopoly had no means of profiting from a given approach, it crushed it. People who prescribed natural medicine were persecuted, and regarding naturally oriented doctors, their licenses were revoked. Schools teaching natural therapies were forced to close. Thus, during the 1930s through 1950s the medical monopolists crushed the natural medicine movement, largely through the powers of government.

At the beginning of the 1900s through the 1930s there were thousands of companies which produced natural medicines. During the depression era some 3500 firms failed. There were simply too many brands, and marketing was poor. Incredibly, as reported by Dennis B. Worthen in his article *The Pharmaceutical Industry, 1902-1952*, profits were low, as were gross sales.

No single company had sales in excess, says Worthen, of, for instance, Macy's in New York City. Then, various vaccines were produced by small manufacturers. Many proved to be contaminated. Worthen further notes that a variety of such vaccines caused sudden death, both in children and adults. What's more, in some children certain vaccines caused tetanus, that is lockjaw. This bears concerns that perhaps many of the original epidemics occurring near or after the turn of the century were due to vaccinations, for instance, the sudden onset of tuberculosis, which is readily transmitted by such injections. In other words, by the injection of unregulated animal secretions into the masses epidemics were created.

During this time private industry created various herbal and natural medicines, which were never endorsed by the government. Medical doctors used such remedies, but the medical system opposed this. In contrast, the government was directly involved with drug houses. In fact, some drug houses were created by government officials.

There was a legitimate reason for government involvement. This was partly due to the fact that such drugs were poisonous. Reports continuously filtered into government offices of fatal reactions to patent medicines. Again, according to Worthen numerous children died as a result of the vaccines, including a constellation of victims—at least five as a result of contaminated diphtheria antitoxin—in St. Louis. Pockets of deaths throughout the country were reported. Apparently, this forced the government's hand. It was decided to regulate this industry, that is the production of potentially deadly serums and inoculations. This was done under what was known as the Public Health Service.

The first license to produce blood-based products commercially was awarded to Parke-Davis and H. K. Mulford. Since then regarding the inoculation business there has been direct government involvement, in fact, control. This is a government procedure and/or business, not a scientific or medical one. To demonstrate the ties as early as 1902 a vested interest was obvious. Government officials, in fact, became connected to the "business of serums." This is demonstrated by the fact that one of America's first producers of vaccines, Lederle Labs, was created by Ernst Joseph Lederle, the former director of the New York Health Department. He was one of the first Americans to receive from the government a license to produce blood- or tissue-related products. Such products are known as biologicals.

The war was a boon for many pharmaceutical companies. Many such companies were run by former government officials. Thus, government contracts were prolific. Blood products became a multimillion dollar business, notably dried plasma. Millions of units of dried plasma were produced. This was fed by the vast blood drives through the war effort established throughout North America. Thirteen pharmaceutical houses were involved in processing blood into dried by-products.

After the war this business essentially ended. The Korean War erupted, but ultimately the need for such blood products declined, causing a vacuum in pharmaceutical sales. Of these wartime companies four were heavily involved in the polio vaccine campaign: Lederle, Wyeth, Parke-Davis, and Cutter. With the loss of military business a national vaccine campaign was a welcome source of income. Further evidence for this need is the fact that during military campaigns vaccine production reaches its height.

During the Korean War a wide range of vaccines were produced and administered. Here, the government 'hires' pharmaceutical houses to produce the desired serums. An entire program was mandated to create antisera and vaccines, as well as various other drugs, to be used in the field. This gave a much needed boost to the drug houses. Contracts were given to such facilities to produce biological weapons. Government officials took posts at such institutions, benefiting from the profits. The weapons were perhaps intended for use in the Korean theater. They were likely used there, yet what is known definitely is that American citizens suffered exposure. Supposed simulations of potential military use were conducted—against Americans. In San Francisco untold billions of dangerous bacteria, notably *Serratia marcesens* and *Bacillus subtilis*, were sprayed from warships from the coast inward. Both are soil-based organisms, which were produced in government-licensed drug houses. Serratia is a type of sewage organism.

Both these bacteria were sprayed directly on humans. What an utter disregard of the human being that such an experiment would be performed. In contrast, it was well known that Serratia is a potential pathogen—during World War II the Germans sprayed it on the English in subways as a biological agent. In fact, in the San Francisco debacle at least one individual died, while numerous others were sickened. Declassified documents indicate that during the military spraying the incidence of respiratory disorders increased 10-fold. In fact, incredibly, Serratia had never before been a serious pathogen. Since its artificial entry into American life it is listed as a major killer, primarily of the hospitalized and the infirm. Some 5,000 to 10,000 deaths yearly are attributed to this germ, mostly from pneumonia. Incredibly, serratia is a biogerm, which has become established in the human population.

In 1953 the Korean War ended. In 1954 the polio vaccine program began. Both were government creations. Both were money-generating operations, fully benefitting the drug cartel. A coincidence is unlikely. There was a need to keep the drug houses busy, to keep pace with the business activity they were accustomed to.

In 1954 the first biological agents were weaponized. This is the same year that the polio vaccine was created.

Its all monkey virus

Simian virus 40 infection is only a part of the dilemma. This is because few people understand this frightening fact: the polio virus itself, the one used to make the vaccine, is to a large degree a monkey virus. It seems the virus, while perhaps originally a human strain, was processed through the tissues of live monkeys to create a supposedly humanoid strain. This processing occurred as early as 1908. The modern strains were derived from these original ones, which were grown in monkeys. Unwittingly the researchers created a combination virus, part ape and human and then used it to produce the vaccine. Usually, before the vaccine virus was harvested to be used as a seed culture, it was inoculated into several types of monkeys. Researchers believed that this would create a strain similar to the human type. They failed to realize that they were creating a kind of freak of nature: a hybrid, part human and part ape. This was the source of the vaccine given to millions of Westerners.

Why did the researchers repeatedly infect monkeys with the virus and then harvest it? The concept was to create a virus that was less likely to cause polio than the native or wild type. Such a virus, it was hoped, would render immunity to the recipient. This was to a degree based upon the fact that it was discovered that once monkeys became infected with polio they developed a seemingly lifelong immunity. Somehow, they were able to live with the virus, without suffering symptoms. Lab operators thought that they could create such a microbe by simply injecting native polio viruses until they became non-infective. Since the virus could live in the monkeys without causing polio, surely, was the thinking, such viruses, if injected into humans, would fail to cause it in them as well. This was the concept upon which mass vaccination was based. It was never fully tested. Thus, rather than proven science it was based upon speculation.

However, lymph is a kind of sacred fluid, and the body makes every attempt to keep it sterile. Lymph saturates every organ in the body. It is directly connected to all fluids, including the venous blood, red blood, cellular fluids, and spinal fluid. Any substance injected into the lymph could contaminate the other fluids. The spinal fluid is particularly vulnerable. This is yet another tyranny of modern vaccines, which introduce a wide range of dangerous substances that gain access, notably through the lymph, to the spinal fluid. The vaccines are injected directly into the lymphatics. This is the job of the lymphatic system: to protect, to absorb, remove, detoxify, and to challenge and purge any invading toxin. Vaccines overload the lymphatic system.

They cause a high degree of toxicity to the thymus, even causing thymic cell destruction. They are also toxic to the bone marrow. Thus, vaccines are a major cause of lymphatic and bone marrow diseases, including lymphoma, lymphedema, neutropenia (that is low white blood cell count), and leukemia.

A persistent disaster

SV40 still exists: in humans. It remains a monumental source of human disease. It systematically infects humans, gradually denuding their health. It is the cause of such vast disease that it is beyond comprehension. Plus, it is readily spread. It is perhaps the most common cause of chronic fatigue syndrome as well as fibromyalgia.

Unless it is aggressively treated, it will likely lead to cancer. New cases are continuously found. Investigators now believe that there was no guarantee that even the latest oral polio immunizations, those given up to the year 2000, when it was discontinued, were safe. These too may have been contaminated with various monkey virus species, including SV40. At a minimum they were contaminated with simian cytomegalovirus, a carcinogenic germ. Even today tumors are being found infested with this virus, even in people born well after the contamination incident.

What's more, according to confidential memos the vaccine's primary maker, Lederle, has admitted it often had no control over the contamination issue and that vaccines, even the ones in use today, may be contaminated. So describes a secretive memo, which confirms that even though their use was prohibited Lederle occasionally used the SV40-carrying rhesus monkeys as a source of cell culture.

No one wants to believe that the government would harm its citizens. What people fail to realize is that the government is only concerned with a single issue: financial interests. Among Americans this trust is virtually universal. Perhaps if everyone realized there truly is no peoples' government and that most government officials are lawyers, this would create a more appropriate perspective. If people regarded the government as a business, only then could they realize its true nature. Only then would they fail to be shocked at government-sponsored tyranny. Only then would they understand the true nature of their own lives—mere pawns to be manipulated by government or, rather, business dictates.

Perhaps the polio shot and/or oral vaccine suppressed the symptoms of polio. Perhaps it forced the disease into remission. Perhaps it prevented pathological cases of the disease. Yet, this doesn't mean it helped the population. It doesn't mean it was a benefit for humankind. It doesn't prove that its benefits outweighed its damage. What's more, the vaccine, as well as various other vaccines, cause polio-like diseases, for instance, Guillain Barré syndrome and Bell's Palsy. The fact is there are tens of thousands of people, rather, millions of them, who have developed damage and disease because of the vaccine.

Many of these individuals have developed a kind of low-grade polio, not enough to paralyze but enough to cause agony. This is essentially subclinical polio caused by the vaccine.

It results in low-level neuromuscular damage, where the vaccine viruses disrupt the function of the body, even partially damaging the brain and spinal cord. It is not the same as paralytic polio, the type where there is obvious paralysis and muscle loss. Rather, it is a slow, systematic destruction, which ultimately renders the individual physically incompetent and barely able to function. Thus, the individual is left with devastated physiology: all due to the neurologically toxic effects of the vaccine—a kind of chronic intracellular polio complicated by noxious carcinogenic animal viruses, including SV40. Such infections cause wasting of the tissues, muscle weakness, and suppressed immunity.

Individuals who are infected with these viruses are virtually constantly ill. Their immune systems are weak, and they readily contract infections. Or, they may suffer from a kind of immune system suppression, where they fail to mount a strong immune response. No longer do they react with a normal immune response: fever, aches, chills, sore throat, etc. They simply become infected, and the immune system fails to react. Fully intoxicated by the vaccine viruses, the body's defense system is incapable of responding to the invader(s), and, as a result, the infections are driven more deeply into the tissues, perpetuating and worsening the condition.

This is the consequence of the polio vaccine. Thus, this cannot be regarded as an award-winning or miraculous cure. Far from a savior for humankind, this vaccine, has caused immeasurable damage, countless deaths, that is from cancer as well as vast numbers of cases of chronic diseases. Even today, because of its toxicity millions of people suffer chronic physical impairment. This vaccine is the cause of several novel diseases, never before known to the human race. Surely, the very medicine which is the cause of devastating epidemics which ravage humankind—surely, it must not also be the cure. The polio vaccine causes the destruction of tissue. In some individuals it causes permanent paralysis. This vaccine has outlived its value if any. The fact is it must be banned from human use.

Modern medicine has failed to cure any disease. Modern vaccinations are, in fact, a cause of disease. Inoculations cause wound syndrome, viral infections, paralysis, autistic disorders, encephalitis, meningitis, multiple sclerosis, autoimmune disorders, and cancer. As a result of this procedure millions of individuals have been stricken with some form of cancer. To this very day hundreds of millions of others suffer the consequences of suppressed immunity. Is this synonymous with a cure?

Why medical people would inject disease-causing germs in an individual is unfathomable. How could the dissemination of disease prevent it? Unfortunately, when noxious substances are dispensed or injected—there will undoubtedly be consequences.

Yet, the original premise of a vaccine is that it is to build immunity—to strengthen the immune system's response against pathogens. This is supposedly so that disease, even death, is prevented. According to Davies' *Infection and Immunity* a vaccine is defined as a "preparation of a pathogen which engenders immunity *without causing disease.*" Regarding today's vaccines that is an oxymoron. All the modern vaccines cause side effects as well as fulminant diseases. All can cause toxic allergic reactions as well as anaphylactic shock. All can potentially cause sudden death. Virtually all have been associated with secondary infections, including neurological infestations. The majority have also been directly connected with the cause of cancer. Thus, by definition all modern vaccines are not true vaccinations. Rather, they are inoculations, which may prevent certain diseases or, rather, repressing the symptoms of such diseases, while causing others.

Yet, the possibility remains that these modern 'vaccines' fail to truly prevent disease, rather, they only prevent symptoms. Likewise, they may cause a germ to go into a repressed state, where such germs cause chronic infections. Thus, they may prevent the symptoms of measles, mumps, and rubella as well as the obvious signs of polio. Yet, a true cure, where all traces of the germs are eradicated, is rarely or never achieved. If vaccines truly worked, for example, there would be a natural immune reaction if the person eventually encountered the germ for measles or mumps. They would experience fever, night sweats, and body aches. This virtually never occurs.

Germs are highly versatile. Injecting germs or germ DNA into the body could never create a cure. Rather, there is always a risk for causing disease. Plus, a germ-filled solution must by nature contain numerous species besides the purported one. In fact, there may be dozens, perhaps hundreds—even thousands—of species of unknown germs in any injection. This is also true of oral vaccines such as the oral polio vaccine. However, while the obvious signs/symptoms may be repressed other not-so-evident disorders fester.

The measles vaccine virus has been found within the human body, where it causes chronic infection. It suppresses the immune system, so that no true measles symptoms occur. Furthermore, it is directly associated with a variety of potentially deadly diseases, including ulcerative colitis, Crohn's disease, and intestinal cancer. Eastern European investigators have determined a connection with this agent and childhood cancer, especially lymphoma and leukemia. Measles rarely kill. Cancer frequently does so. Plus, it causes untold agony and misery. The trade-off is poor.

It is bad enough to inject disease-causing organisms into the body or, in the case of the oral polio vaccine, ingest them. By nature disease-causing organisms are dangerous: they cannot be handled or consumed with absolute safety. That is why they are called pathogens: they are pathogenic, meaning disease-causing. This is why such extreme measures must be taken when dealing with them—they must be treated with the most harsh chemicals to render them even partially 'safe'. These formidable chemicals include chlorinated compounds, benzene, mercurial compounds, formaldehyde (embalming fluid), and irradiation. Such substances/procedures are themselves toxic. What's more, these treatment procedures create harsh by-products, such as chlorinated hydrocarbons, mutated germs, mutated genetic material, and cell wall-deficient germs, the latter being fully able to infect.

All such by-products can cause illness and disease. No vaccine company can prove that such substances are safe. Nor can they prove that these substances or procedures fail to cause disease. The fact is there is a plethora of evidence proving that they, in fact, do cause disease.

The vaccine industry has changed little since it began, some 110 years ago. Animal products are used to grow microbes, primarily viruses. The resulting fluids, which include blood residues, are 'harvested' causing a horrible death to living animals, and the drug is created. Once the virus solution is created, it is minimally processed, which increases the risks for disease transmission. Usually, no heat is used—the germs are neutralized with harsh chemicals, perhaps radiation. Thus, a vaccine is truly a blood product, in some cases a raw one, and it contains all the various substances, as well as germs, which would be expected to exist in that blood. The type of blood derivatives found in vaccines is dependent upon the growth medium: bovine, poultry, porcine, canine, simian, murine (that is mouse), equine (that is horse), and even human. Yes, a wide range of cell sources are used.

Few people realize that every vaccine introduces a different kind of blood. This is a treatment which violates most religions. The Torah, Bible, and Qur'an all prohibit the consumption of blood. In this regard the Qur'an and Torah are clear; they also prohibit the consumption of pork, claiming the meat as (microbially) filthy. Even if the vaccine components are supposedly dead, still, it is blood tissue. No doubt, whether dead, partially alive, or alive, it remains active, that is immunologically. The immune system regards foreign blood products as the enemy. It will raise combat against them. This is the premise of vaccines. However, there is no guarantee that this combat will be beneficial. Again, vaccines are based on a theory. They have never been proven to be safe nor are they proven to be effective.

In epidemics vaccines may offer benefit. These vaccines must be made directly from the epidemic germ and must only be used until the crisis is quelled. In daily life in civilized cultures they have proven disastrous. Consider the diseases directly related to modern vaccines: autism, attention deficit syndrome, multiple sclerosis, Parkinson's disease, Alzheimer's disease, ankylosing spondylitis, nephritis, pericarditis, Guillain-Barré syndrome, autoimmune thyroid disease, and Addison's disease. Yet, this is only a partial list. It is not a matter of a trade-off. It is a modern catastrophe. The administration of such agents made from disease-bearing animal blood must be halted immediately. This is the only way Americans can readily achieve excellent health.

The entire concept of vaccination begets danger. There are two main types of vaccines: the so-called inactivated type, which the public presumes is dead, and the type known as attenuated. It is defined as "to weaken." Attenuation is based upon a theory, that if a germ accommodates long enough within a host, then it becomes non-infective. Perhaps this is so in the case of actively obvious symptoms. The caveat is that no one considered the long term consequences, that is the fact that many such attenuated germs are carcinogenic. Who is to say that, perhaps, the altered virus is any safer than the wild type? This means that rather than causing a sudden infection, complete with the expected symptoms, rather, they cause a chronic smoldering infestation, which leads to degenerative diseases, particularly cancer.

Consider why it is so rare for people today to have a strong immune system and to react properly, perhaps violently, to an infection with fever, chills, aches, and prostration. It is largely a consequence of the vaccinations that such an immune response is rare.

The vaccine industry is based upon guesswork. Scientific facts play little if any role. There is no proof that vaccines perform to their claim, which is to cause an overall improvement in public health. Rather, there is evidence documenting the opposite. Actually, they add burdens to public health, in fact, causing an irreparable decline in peoples' health.

Had the public known that the original virus, or father germ was developed in monkeys, that it wasn't merely a human polio virus but, rather, a hybrid freak of nature, part ape and part human, there would have been more resistance. No one was informed of this fact. Had people only known, particularly in the scientific community, including doctors, the resistance would have been fierce. Many Americans would have rejected the vaccines. A protest would have been launched. All this was hidden from the public, fully to their loss and destruction.

Direct evidence

Viruses are capable of causing cancer. This has been known for decades. In his work in Africa the British researcher Burkitt proved that certain viruses can cause liver and lymphatic cancer. Here, the virus is virtually the sole cause of the cancer. In other words, without the viral infection the cancer would fail to develop. The involved virus is Epstein-Barr, a kind of herpetic virus. The disease it causes is known as Hodgkin's lymphoma.

Cancer cells are abnormal, that is their genetic machinery is abnormal. This lends to a viral cause. This is because viruses invade not just the cell but, more importantly, the cell nucleus. Here, they directly attack the nuclear material, splicing their genetic material into the cell's. This means that, genetically, the cell is part human and part virus. The virus now controls the cell's function, even its purpose. Thus, it can be readily understood how the virus creates cancer. Without the virus there would be no cancer. Thus, the virus is the cause.

Viruses reproduce wildly. They create out-of-control infections. According to W. M. Stanley in his book *Viruses and The Nature of Life* "Cancer begins when an apparently normal cell...undergoes a change, which causes it to reproduce *wildly*." This surely implies a viral cause. Stanley continues, "Cancerous tissue is marked not by the great speed with which the cells multiply but by the fact that cell reproduction is *uncontrolled*." This is a critical finding. This is why cancer must not be feared. It won't kill overnight. The tumor grows in an uncontrolled fashion, but not usually exceptionally rapidly. It is a slow bizarre growth, an instigation in the tissues. If the instigator can be purged, that is if the cause can be removed, then, the tumor growth will be halted, in other words the tumor will die.

The insensibility of fear is illustrated by another fact mentioned by Stanley: that, incredibly, normal tissues, including the cells of the liver and intestinal lining, grow more rapidly than most cancer. This is the debacle of the orthodox cancer treatments, radiation and chemotherapy, both of which destroy such fast-growing tissues.

There is another fact which is rarely discussed. Cancer is always surrounded by normal tissues. Thus, not all tissues are diseased. There is a locale of disease: something within these tissues is provoking, creating, the tumor—something is stimulating the growth, directly in that area. It can't be the cell—there is something within the cell that is responsible. If it was the cells, then, all the cells of the area would be cancerous. Thus, again, there is a toxic reaction within the tumor, which is specific to that region. The toxin may arise from elsewhere, but the fact remains that the local area is diseased—it cannot be due merely to abnormal cell growth. There must be a provocative factor, and it is most likely viral.

Viruses overtake the cellular machinery. In some instances the genetic materials are fully usurped. Only viruses can achieve this. The fact is this is how they cause cancers. Other microbes may influence the genes, notably fungi. Yet, it is viruses alone which can take full control of the cellular operations, directing the cells to perform their bidding by causing the cells to produce viral material. Fungi also can alter the cells' genetics. However, it is viruses which if uncontested completely leverage the cellular machinery, even if that means the creation of tumors. Tumors encourage viral growth, while healthy cells block it. Thus, the virus's entire purpose is to create disease, in fact, cancer. This is true of no other microbe.

The gall on a plant—that bulbous, distorted growth which disfigures and, in fact, corrupts it is due to a virus. By nature viruses are tumor-causing. If they infect the body, it is expected that they also create growths. Fungi also cause gall-like lesions, so they too are tumor-producing. The combination of viral and fungal infectious could prove deadly.

Persistent viral infections dramatically increase the risks for tumor formation. What's more, viruses infect the body via stealth. This means that even though they are damaging the body they may not cause noticeable symptoms. It is their purpose to evade detection, so they can survive. Once within the cell, they overtake the genetic functions, fully controlling cellular destiny. Deep within the cell they may evade detection for decades, while systematically damaging the tissues.

This is the ideal mechanism for cancer formation: the slow, advancing distortion, which proceeds continuously without symptoms for years. Or, the symptoms are so minimal that they are difficult to pinpoint, perhaps ignored. No doctor can find the cause: it is an undetectable viral infection, which if left uncorrected, will result in cancer. Thus, the virus must be purged from the body. This is the only means for the cure.

There is no need for deadly chemicals as cancer cures. All that is needed is to destroy the stealth viruses. This will cause the reversal of the majority of cancers. Surely, there are other causes of cancer besides viruses. Toxic chemicals initiate this disease. They do so by damaging the genes, thereby weakening the cells and organs. Yet, this is the ideal environment for viral invasion. Whenever the internal powers of the cells are weakened, whenever the cell walls are damaged or the genetics chemically altered—this is when viruses gain a foothold.

It is much easier for viruses to invade damaged tissue than if they are healthy. Toxic chemicals that are responsible for cancer, such as pesticides, fungicides, herbicides, chlorinated compounds, fluorinated compounds, gasoline derivatives, alcohol, and solvents, also damage the immune system. Many such chemicals outright destroy the immune components: the lymphatic tissues, bone marrow, and white cells. Drugs also do this.

A number of pharmaceutical drugs directly damage the bone marrow, which is responsible for the production of white blood cells. Drugs which exert this toxicity include antibiotics, cortisone, Prednisone, and chemotherapeutic agents. Vaccines are also notorious for damaging the immune system. They exert direct toxicity against the lymphatic tissues as well as bone marrow. Repeated vaccinations are a primary cause of a reduced immune response and, particularly, a lowered white blood cell count. In any individual with a low white blood cell count for which no obvious cause can be found vaccines must be suspected as the culprit. The lowered white blood cell count in recipients of multiple vaccines is a clear sign of the great toxicity of these injections. Radiation also damages the immune system and is particularly toxic to the bone marrow. Stanley fully demonstrates the dangers of radiation, a known cause of cancer. Yet, what he reveals is even more insidious.

Medical professionals have rejected the role of viruses in cancer, that is a universal role. The official position is that only 30% of human cancers are infective. Yet, this is a considerable number, which demonstrates that of all known causes infection predominates.

The reason for the lack of acceptance of the infection theory dates to the late 1800s. This is because the majority of researchers hold to an original theory published over a century ago by the German investigator Koch. According to Koch's theory if infection is truly the cause of cancer, then, if cancerous tissue is injected into test animals, the animal will become noticeably infected with the disease. There will be a direct transfer, Koch believed, with matching symptoms.

This is the sole basis for the rejection of the infection connection to cancer. Yet, regarding Koch and his followers no account was taken for the long-term consequences of such an injection, that is the potential for cancer development years later. In most cancers if the cancerous tissue is tested by injecting it into a test subject, usually, no obvious infections or even cancers develop. Even so, in some instances fulminant disease quickly strikes. However, usually, it takes years for cancer to develop, so there is no way to truly assess the toxicity of germ-laden injections. As described by Stanley "appearances (can) deceive." This is because, he notes, viruses are fully capable of operating within tissue "without exhibiting the usual signs of infection." This essentially nullifies the Koch theory. Thus, potentially most all cancers may have a microbial origin.

Such organisms slowly and methodically infect human cells, fully cannibalizing them—fully overwhelming them. This occurs with few if any symptoms, certainly no symptoms of acute disease such as fever, chills, and sore throat. There may be symptoms, but they are hardly distinguishable: fatigue, sluggish mental function, and a sensation of not feeling 100%. Rarely, there may be night sweats and a slight fever. Usually, there are no noticeable "infective" symptoms. Stanley further notes that the "concealed virus" persists in infecting the tissue at a low level and that a sudden stress may reveal it. Here, it was found that if the cells are traumatized by a sudden stressor—the toxicity from exposure to a chemical, drug, or, particularly, radiation, the virus goes out of bounds. It becomes transformed from a smoldering parasite to a violent invader, a diabolical opportunist, decimating all in its path. It takes advantage of the weakened state of the organism by cannibalizing it.

Radiation also traumatizes the tissues, increasing the invasiveness of viruses. What's more, it increases the invasive powers of fungi, since radiation creates numerous bizarre mutants. When cells are exposed to significant doses of radiation, mutated germs are created which can attack the tissues. Radiation greatly increases the fungi's infective powers. What's more, it is directly toxic to cells, that is the cell structures are weakened to such a degree that viral, as well as fungal, infections readily develop.

Growing wildly, it systematically destroys the body. This demonstrates how deadly the combination of the viral infection plus toxic stress really is. The body's defenses are strong, but if they are broken, then, there is only utter mayhem. Thus, any antiviral campaign must combine two methods: the systematic destruction of the virus plus the strengthening of the cellular defenses.

The polio virus itself is carcinogenic. It is a stool virus—it should never be injected into the body. Even if killed, it is toxic, as would be expected from a fecal germ. Thus, whether by injection or oral intake exposure to the polio virus can only lead to disease. The fact is this is true of any stool pathogen.

There is no sound medical basis for such an approach. To put people at risk with such an injection or an oral dose is inconceivable: especially with a known pathogen. Germs cause disease. To avoid disease the normal approach is to avoid such germs. How can infecting the body with them improve health? This doesn't even make sense. The injections, as well as oral vaccine, are given repeatedly. It is a kind of toxic bombardment with either dead germs, germ genetic material, inactivated germs, or living germs. Only harm could result from such a toxicity. The body cannot be burdened with such a microbial load without suffering damage.

Routinely, vaccines suppress the immune system. This is largely due to the antigenic load. What's more, they introduce a plethora of chemicals, many of which are carcinogenic. Furthermore, today, vaccines are genetically engineered, which introduces a host of further problems. With such a vast potential for toxic reactivity within the body it is no surprise that vaccines can cause sudden death. Shock reactions immediately after vaccinations are common. Yearly, hundreds of individuals, including infants and children, die from such reactions. This is indisputable. The FDA has such records on file.

The Sabin/Salk vaccine is the greatest catastrophe of all, because this contamination created specific diseases never before known. Yet, it also is a major cause of the global cancer epidemic, which afflicts Western peoples. Bizarre cancers never before known developed after the introduction of these vaccines. These reduced the human race to become contaminated with a man-made monkey virus known to cause cancer.

The fact that tens of millions of Westerners have developed this infection is difficult to dispute. This raises the question of just who is infected. It is possible to determine the degree of infection through symptom analysis. There is no blood test for this disorder. Only symptom analysis can reveal it. Such an evolution is crucial, since by determining early infection corrective action can be taken.

The proper treatment, which largely consists of wild spice extracts such as Oreganol P73 along with food-like germ killers, for instance, cold-pressed garlic oil and oil of propolis, can be prescribed. Such a treatment plan will save innumerable lives and prevent untold misery. This is because death by mad cow syndrome is among the most gruesome forms of agony known. This is a man-made disease. Thus, there is no reason to lose hope. Aggressive treatment with spice oils, as well as the important water soluble spice extract Oreganol Juice of Oregano, will save lives. The Oreganol juice crosses the blood-brain barrier. Plant flavonoids are also invaluable, as are aromatic flower essences.

Monkey virus symptom test

This test provides an accurate assessment of the relatively difficult-to-diagnose simian virus 40 infection. There is no common blood test for this condition. Thus, it is the symptoms that are the most reliable check, as is demonstrated by the following:

CASE HISTORY:

Ms. T. called me on the radio, complaining about various symptoms. I immediately became suspicious of SV40 syndrome. While on the air I said she must be between 50 and 60 years old, which proved correct. This confirmed that she was a recipient of the various monkey virus-contaminated polio vaccines. I then asked her if she had the cardinal symptoms of SV40 infection: numbness and tingling, fatigue, exhaustion, numbness in her fingers, and spinal stiffness. She confirmed all such symptoms. Then, I demanded, she must have been given the oral sugar cube vaccine (that is the Sabin vaccine), which she confirmed. She was instructed to take the wild oregano (P73) purge. Within three months she experienced a major increase in energy, plus a significant improvement in all other symptoms.

Answer all of the following questions and calculate the score. Which of these applies to you?

Signs/symptoms	Points

1. numbness and tingling . . . .(2)
2. loss of muscular strength . . . .(2)
3. loss of sensation . . . .(2)
4. loss of the size of muscles, usually on one
    side of the body . . . .(3)
5. spinal stiffness . . . .(2)
6. chronic headaches, unrelieved by medication . . . .(1)
7. leukemia . . . .(3)
8. pituitary disorders or tumors . . . .(2)
9. multiple sclerosis . . . .(4)
10. ALS (that is Lou Gehrig's disease) . . . .(5)
11. brain tumor . . . .(5)
12. mesothelioma . . . .(10)
13. bone cancer . . . .(3)
14. stiff neck . . . .(1)
15. immune deficiency . . . .(3)
16. low white blood count . . . .(2)
17. low amount of blood proteins . . . .(2)
18. bone marrow disorders, including low platelet count .(3)
19. numbness in the bottoms of the feet . . . .(1)
20. frequent herpetic outbreaks
    (shingles, genital herpes, etc.) . . . .(2)
21. severe cold sores . . . .(2)
22. unusual mouth ulcers . . . .(1)
23. epileptic seizures . . . .(3)
24. spastic muscles . . . .(3)
25. persistent tremors . . . .(2)
26. chronic fatigue syndrome . . . .(2)

27. fibromyalgia ....(2)
28. polymyositis rheumatica ....(3)
29. persistent spastic colon or irritable bowel syndrome . .(2)
30. Crohn's disease and/or ulcerative colitis ....(2)
31. failure to thrive ....(1)
32. benign growths throughout the body ....(3)
33. persistent asthma ....(1)
34. thin frail body type ....(1)
35. swelling of the lower legs ....(1)
36. constantly sick as a child ....(3)
37. tumors of the kidneys ....(3)
38. nephritis ....(3)
39. polycystic kidney disease ....(2)
40. systemic lupus ....(2)
41. psychosis ....(2)
42. schizophrenia ....(2)
43. anxiety-neurosis ....(2)
44. mental retardation ....(5)
45. sluggish kidney function ....(1)
46. kidney failure ....(2)
47. muscular dystrophy ....(4)
48. myasthenia gravis ....(2)
49. autoimmune disorders ....(2)
50. encephalitis of unknown origin ....(3)
51. paralysis ....(3)
52. immune system highly sluggish ....(2)
53. persistent tiredness ....(1)
54. spinal muscles are spastic ....(2)
55. dysfunctional child ....(2)
56. muscular uncoordination ....(2)
57. Parkinson's disease ....(3)
58. cerebral palsy-like disease ....(3)
59. muscles are weak or poor muscular tone ....(1)

60. when sick, rarely mount a fever response . . . .(2)
61. autoimmune thyroid disorder . . . .(4)
62. adrenal disorder . . . .(3)
63. pituitary disorder or growth . . . .(3)
64. sudden blindness (as a child) . . . .(2)
65. sudden loss of vision or visual impairment
    (as a child or teenager) . . . .(2)
66. sudden development of arthritis
    (as a child or teenager) . . . .(3)
67. lymphoma (non-Hodgkins) . . . .(10)
68. lymphatic cancer (any other type) . . . .(5)
69. sudden weight gain during childhood,
    cause unknown . . . .(2)
70. sudden development during childhood of diabetes . . .(3)
71. neuropathy . . . .(2)
72. foot drop or major loss of muscle tissue on one side . .(2)
73. severe exhaustion . . . .(1)
74. infection of the brain or brain stem (cause unknown) .(5)
75. pemphigus or other bulbous skin disorders . . . .(2)

Your score _____

2 to 8 points Mild SV40/stealth virus infection:

Stealth monkey viruses could be a major factor of your health problems. There is no truly mild case possible. There may be other factors, such as chronic fungal infections or infections by other viruses such as cytomegalovirus and Epstein-Barr. For prevention take oil of wild oregano, five drops twice daily. Take also the crude wild oregano capsules, that is the OregaMax crude herbal capsules, three capsules twice daily. Even at this level to avoid the development of an SV40-induced tumor a wild oregano purge is necessary. See the Purge Protocol (Appendix A).

9 to 19 points Moderate SV40/stealth virus infection:

The likelihood for stealth viral infection is high. There may be other complicating factors such as infections by other viruses, such as cytomegalovirus, Epstein-Barr, and HIV. There could also be fungal and/or parasitic infections, perhaps chronic bacterial invasion. Regardless, a purge using the wild oregano extracts would prove invaluable. Take the oil of wild oregano (P73 blend), ten to twenty drops twice daily. Take also the OregaBiotic, two or more capsules twice daily. To aid in eradicating viral invasion of the nervous system take the Juice of wild Oregano, one ounce twice daily. Also, see the Purge Protocol (Appendix A).

20 to 30 points Severe SV40/stealth virus infection:

The likelihood for stealth viral infection is exceptionally high. There may be other complicating factors such as infections by other viruses, for instance, simian cytomegalovirus, Epstein-Barr, retroviruses and HIV. There could also be fungal and/or parasitic infections, perhaps chronic bacterial invasion. Regardless, a purge using the wild oregano extracts would prove invaluable. Take the oil of wild oregano (P73 SuperStrength), twenty or more drops twice daily (or use the capsules). Take also the OregaBiotic, three or more capsules twice daily. Even the monkey stealth viruses will be purged under such power. To aid in eradicating viral invasion of the nervous system take the Juice of wild Oregano, one or more ounces twice daily. Take also the highly aromatic Neuroloft, one ounce twice daily. The PropaHeal (that is oil of propolis), is a potent virucide: take one-half dropperful twice daily. As a natural antiinflammatory take the Inflam-eez, two capsules twice daily on an empty stomach and wait one hour before eating. Also, see the Purge Protocol (Appendix A).

31 to 50 points Extreme SV40/stealth virus infection:

Warning, stealth viruses have invaded your body and are placing you at risk for serious diseases, particularly autoimmune disorders, diabetes, heart disease, and cancer. Besides the monkey viruses there may be other complicating factors such as infections by other viruses, like cytomegalovirus, Epstein-Barr, retrovirus and HIV. There could also be fungal and/or parasitic infections, perhaps chronic bacterial invasion. Regardless, a purge using the wild oregano extracts would prove invaluable. Take the oil of wild oregano (P73 SuperStrength), two droppersful twice daily (or use the capsules). Also, on a daily basis rub the SuperStrength up and down the spine, and take OregaBiotic, three or more capsules twice daily on an empty stomach and wait one hour before eating. Take also the Inflam-eez two capsules three times daily. In the case of respiratory symptoms take also two OregaRESP.

Even the monkey stealth viruses will be purged under such power. To help eradicate viral invasion of the nervous system take the Juice of wild Oregano, two or more ounces twice daily. Take also the highly aromatic Juice of Rosemary, one ounce twice daily. Also, take the highly aromatic Neuroloft, one or more ounces twice daily. For additional antiseptic power take the Garlex cold-pressed garlic oil, two or more droppersful twice daily. The PropaHeal (that is oil of wild propolis, North American Herb & Spice), is a potent virucide: take one dropperful twice daily. Also, be sure to eat a high protein diet, and strictly avoid the intake of legumes, particularly peanuts and beans, as well as chocolate.

Absolutely no chocolate or alcohol may be consumed. Also, see the Purge Protocol (Appendix A). With such high doses of spice extracts take also a natural healthy bacterial supplement, for instance, Health-Bac. Ideally, take a half teaspoon of the Health-Bac in warm water at bedtime.

51 points and above Profoundly Extreme SV40/stealth virus infection:

Warning, you are suffering from a dangerous degree of stealth virus invasion. Your risk for the development of stealth virus-induced cancer and autoimmune diseases is monumentally high. Without treatment a stealth virus-induced cancer will assuredly develop. Besides the monkey viruses there may be other complicating factors such as infections by cytomegalovirus, Epstein-Barr, retrovirus and HIV: there could also be fungal and/or parasitic infections, perhaps chronic bacterial invasion. At all costs aggressively purge from your body these viruses. This can be achieved by taking the wild oregano extracts in large doses. Take the oil of wild oregano (P73 SuperStrength), four droppersful twice daily (or use the capsules). Also, on a daily basis rub the SuperStrength up and down the spine. Take also the OregaBiotic, three or more capsules four times daily.

Even the monkey stealth viruses will be purged under such power. To help eradicate viral invasion of the nervous system take the Juice of wild Oregano, two or more ounces twice daily. Also, take the Neuroloft, two ounces twice daily Take also the highly aromatic Juice of Rosemary, two or more ounces twice daily. For additional antiseptic power take the Garlex cold-pressed garlic oil, two or more droppersful twice daily. In addition, take the Inflam-eez, two capsules three or more times daily. The PropaHeal (that is oil of propolis, North American Herb & Spice), is a potent virucide: take one or two droppersful twice daily. Also, be sure to eat a high protein diet, and strictly avoid the intake of legumes, particularly peanuts and beans, as well as chocolate. Absolutely no chocolate or alcohol should be consumed. Also, see the Purge Protocol in Appendix A.

Untreated, SV40 will likely lead to cancer. The germ is difficult to eradicate. A purge is only part of the answer. There must also be a maintenance effort, that is where the appropriate supplements are taken on a daily basis. It is primarily the wild oregano oil—the P73 edible blend—that must be routinely consumed, along with the OregaBiotic. These formulas alone are sufficient to prevent SV40-induced catastrophes. For the neurological component the Oreganol Juice and the Neuroloft are ideal. There is an aberrant growth in human bodies. If this growth is neglected—if no attempt is made to stem it or eradicate it—only catastrophe will result. Natural medicines are the only hope for resolution. There will never be a drug to resolve this condition. The fact is this disease was created by drug vaccine therapy.

Natural medicines boost immunity. Certain of such medicines, notably the spice oils, are invaluable germicides. It is such oils which are capable of eradicating from the tissues stealth invaders such as the notorious SV40. Antioxidants are also invaluable, that is for protecting cellular tissues. Wild oregano, the active ingredient of the Oreganol, as well as cumin and sage, among the most potent antioxidants known.

Natural medicines boost immunity, while healing and preserving the tissues. By taking the appropriate natural medicines the dangerous effects of the monkey stealth viruses can be minimized, perhaps eliminated. That is the best option available, since, regarding this disease there is no medical cure.

SV40 is a crime against humanity. There is no possibility that such a disease could become established naturally. It had to be imposed upon the people by criminal men, who sought only personal gain. The fact is SV40 and all off its consequences are created by medicine itself. What's more, there is no medical cure. Could there be any greater tyranny than that?

Chapter 6
Dangerous Medicine

Live viruses are dangerous. Most vaccines contain them. Such viruses should never be injected into the body. Even if the viruses are genetically or chemically altered, that is weakened, still, they should not be injected.

Clearly, as a result of these injections there is a risk for damage, particularly in individuals with weak or vulnerable systems. According to *Infection and Immunity* in people with sluggish or depressed immune systems, for instance, those taking medications, chemotherapy, radiation, or who simply have an immunological disease, if a live vaccine is given, the viruses might "replicate with impunity." This is particularly true in those with immune deficiencies, including AIDS victims, hepatitis patients, and those with asthma, psoriasis, and/or eczema. The authors also note that there is a risk that the virus might invade and infect the brain, which clearly demonstrates how aggressive and dangerous these organisms are. It also demonstrates the fallacy of attempting to cure disease through the ingestion or injection of these agents. Thus, could various neurological diseases be due primarily to invasive viruses or viral genetic material originating from vaccinations? Only further research will tell.

All vaccines are dangerous. This is true even of the rabies vaccine, which is one of the few which saves lives. Even so, the vaccinated live an agonizing existence, largely due to the toxicity of the therapy. Anyone who receives rabies vaccines should simultaneously take spice oil extracts, such as wild oil of Oreganol, as a support.

The rabies vaccine has an interesting history. Originally, it was made by Pasteur, who produced the vaccine virus in the brains of rabbits. The spinal cords of infected rabbits were then dried, which reduced the virulence of the virus. Even so, among the recipients autoimmune paralysis, nerve disorders, brain inflammation, agitation, depression, psychosis, muscular diseases, and arthritic symptoms were common.

Modern vaccines are produced from highly contaminated materials, for instance, human placenta, dog kidney, monkey kidney, and chicken embryo. All such tissues are infested with a wide range of germs.

With vaccines made from such sources the simultaneous use of the wild oregano extract is crucial. This is particularly true regarding any vaccine made from human tissue, such as the human rabies vaccine, since there is a risk of transmitting potentially fatal germs, including the mad cow agent. Since it is a common practice to give certain high risk individuals, such as kennel workers, the vaccine preventively, such individuals should consider the daily intake of wild oregano extract (Oreganol P73). This is a potent antiviral agent and, in fact, potentiates the effectiveness of the vaccine. In humans and in cell cultures it destroys pathogenic viruses.

Regarding the actions of the vaccines, that is the theory of how they supposedly work, researchers are unsure of "what constitutes an effective protective immune response." In other words, the researchers/manufacturers are aware that vaccines exert an action upon the immune system, but they are unable to demonstrate if it is effective or perhaps ineffective. It was again the authors of *Infection and Immunity* who revealed that "conventional vaccines have been made by trial and error, without any real understanding of the virulence of the pathogen." What an incredible admission it is: it is as if to say, "We don't really know what we are doing, but we hope it works."

Clearly, at a minimum this means that this approach is unscientific as well as unproven. It would appear that the proponents of modern medicine themselves admit that their wares are haphazard. If they are unscientific, as well as unsafe, why take them? The fact is with aggressive therapy, such as saturation of the wound site with SuperStrength oil of wild oregano and its persistent internal intake, for instance, 10 or 20 drops every few minutes, rabies can be treated without vaccinations.

Now an even more unscientific approach is being taken, again based upon guesswork. This involves the creation of genetically engineered viruses. There is no scientific basis for such vaccines. These are truly experimental, without proof of safety or use other than evil intent.

What is in vaccines?

By nature vaccines are contaminated. These contaminants are injected into the blood, where they cause toxic reactions. The reactions and toxicity extend into the organs. Here is where the most profound damage can occur. With all vaccines the toxic elements quickly enter the blood stream as well as the lymphatics. Here, they wreak havoc, provoking inflammation, invading cells, and disrupting cellular function. Thus, vaccines are a systemic agent, in fact, a full body poison, which directly and harshly acts upon the internal organs, including the brain.

These are animal-derived serums. They are also germ cultures. The cultured fluid is the major component of the vaccine. It is the culture medium which makes them so dangerous as well as any chemicals used in the process. Plus, vaccines contain various animal-source proteins, as well as the proteins of dead, partially dead, and living germs. Such substances fully contaminate the body. There can be no doubt about it: it is impossible to inject these proteins into the body without causing toxicity. The proteins are foreign: even if they are "treated" or "attenuated" the body will react to them, often violently. Thus, clearly, this type of therapy causes a greater degree of toxicity than any benefit. This is because the injection of such a wide array of proteins, animal-derived materials, germs, and germ residues will violently damage the body, particularly the immune system. The immune system will become overloaded. The fact is it will become overwhelmed with attempting to purge such a load.

The immune system on its own is incapable of destroying SV40 and similar vaccine viruses. To purge these organisms it requires significant assistance. The introduction of monkey virus components dramatically depresses immunity. The immune system becomes so consumed with reversing the toxicity it is unable to perform its primary job: to protect the body from sudden invaders. Plus, various animal-source germs, such as the SV40, are fully capable of causing the destruction of critical immune components, for instance, bone marrow cells and white blood cells. SV40 has one goal: to utterly corrupt the immune system.

Cynthia Cournoyer notes in her heavily referenced book, *What About Immunizations: Exposing the Vaccine Philosophy*, that vaccine manufacturers themselves know the vaccines are toxic. This was also confirmed by a former FDA chief virologist, J. Anthony Morris, M.D., who was, in fact, fired due to his statements. Yet, no effort is made to protect the public from the danger. According to Cournoyer:

> Vaccines contain killed or diluted infectious agents, solutions containing toxins of these organisms, or substances extracted from infectious agents. Animal parts, such as pig or horse blood, dog kidney tissue, monkey kidney tissue, chicken or duck egg protein, and other decomposing proteins, are used to grow the viruses. In the early 1970s a vaccine researcher, Leonard Hayflick, warned against the use of monkey tissue in the production of polio vaccines. The SV40 virus...was found in the polio vaccine. The problem of virus contamination of monkeys was once so bad that 60% to 80% of monkeys used to make polio vaccine had to be rejected (yet) most of the world's polio vaccine is still made from kidney tissue of African green monkeys and rhesus macaques.

Medical hazard: the danger of foreign protein

At any time the injection of animal protein—the protein found in the blood of, for instance, hogs, horses, chicken, ducks, cats, and dogs—is hazardous. It is well known that the sudden introduction of such proteins into the blood elicits a potent immune reaction, which is systemic. This is because it is the immune system's job to attack such proteins as foreign. This is the basis of allergy testing, for instance, the ELISA or scratch tests. Here, a foreign protein is either complexed on a slide with blood or injected into the skin. Regarding the latter the reaction can be visually measured—a toxic protein creates an inflammatory reaction and the size of the skin lesion tells of the degree of allergy.

This demonstrates what happens internally when the body is exposed to such a protein. Obviously, the same occurs with vaccinations, in fact, more so. This is because allergy testing attempts to demonstrate what happens to the body after a potentially toxic protein is consumed, either through eating or the breathing. When such a protein is injected, it is entirely different. The increase in toxicity is far greater. The toxic protein, in fact, fails to "stimulate" the immune system, rather, it destroys it. It was Nandan who showed through careful blood testing that when foreign or allergenic proteins are ingested, there is no boosting of the immune system. Rather, there is immune system, as well as blood cell, damage. He demonstrated that even the ingestion of common food proteins causes cell death, notably the death of white and red blood cells. It can only be imagined the scope of the damage that results from the injection of animal protein from the chicken, duck, pig, cow, calf, mouse, human, and/or monkey. This is why vaccines can cause sudden shock, even death.

The injection of such proteins could never be deemed safe. The fact is, globally, every year thousands of individuals die from vaccine reactions. Says Courneyer:

> Besides the risk of transferring animal viruses to humans...one must consider...the danger of injecting animal proteins. Proteins by themselves cannot be used by the body. They must be broken down during the digestive process into amino acids before they can be taken into the bloodstream...If any protein enters the bloodstream by any means other than the digestive tract, it becomes a strong poison.

It was Richard Rhodes in his book *Deadly Feasts* who demonstrated the danger of injection versus the oral route. Quoting research by neurobiologist, Frank O. Bastian, M. D., he claimed that the risk of spreading disease, particularly neurological infections, is some one million times greater with systemic invasion such as occurs during vaccinations than with ingestion. For instance, it is well known that despite contamination of the commercial meat supply the primary way of contracting mad cow disease, known medically as Cruetzfeldt-Jakob disease, rather than through ingestion is through contaminated surgical instruments. Apparently, these surgical instruments are contaminated with residues of human brain tissue, which is the source of the infection. Brain tissue is sticky; it is difficult to completely cleanse it from instruments. If this tissue enters the body, mad cow disease can result. Thus, the direct introduction of animal-source protein, as well as brain tissue, is a primary cause of human disease. These tissues contain unknown germs, which can cause potentially fatal diseases.

Mad cow-like agents are likely introduced through vaccinations. This is because the contamination of the vaccines by neurological tissue cannot be ruled out. What's more, the very blood and cell tissue which are used to grow the viruses are usually contaminated. This contamination is from tainted commercial feed which affects the tissue and blood of the pigs, cows, calves, ducks, chickens, and horses that are used to grow the vaccine cultures. Surely, regarding the chicken and duck eggs used for viral growth, these are derived from commercial sources. What's more, the commercial poultry are fed the residues of rendered meat scraps, which are rife with mad cow-like agents. Such agents thrive in the blood of these animals, and if that blood is used as a growth medium for the vaccines, then, the vaccines will be contaminated. So will anyone who is injected with them.

The additives in vaccines are no minor issue. The fact is vaccines contain some of the most toxic chemicals known. Such chemicals include heavy metals, particularly mercury and aluminum, solvents, for instance, acetone, and antibiotics. No one would knowingly allow such chemicals/heavy metals to be injected into the body. In any dose mercury is highly poisonous. When injected, this toxicity is greatly increased.

Obviously, the drug companies know that such vaccines are poisonous. Vaccine lobbyists push for government contracts, which are worth hundreds of millions, even billions, of dollars. Safety is the least concern. How else could there be a government mandate to take medicines containing known poisons, including documented neurotoxins capable of destroying brain tissue? The fact is it has been known for decades that small amounts of mercury, such as the amounts found in childhood vaccines, cause brain damage. Companies sell this mercury to the vaccine cartel. In fact, it is the drug companies which largely make these poisons. Such a source must be investigated for a conflict of interest, in fact, fraud. This is because the injection in infants and children of mercurial compounds is a major cause of disease as well as death. It would appear that vaccines are purposely turned into poisons—what other conclusion could there be?

The vaccine makers seemingly have an utter disregard for human health. They fail to ensure human safety. Such companies have no safety data to prove that for any age group their wares are safe. On the contrary they have evidence that their productions are harmful, even toxic. What's more, the vaccine makers are fully aware that there is a risk for fatality. Thus, profits are their only concern. The fact is they are busy covering up the side effects of their wares. Rather than public concern it is the greed and lust for money which drives them.

What else could explain their method, to use the blood of animals, many of which are knowingly diseased, to create 'medicines'? What else could explain the willing use of poisonous substances, including mercury, aluminum, ethylene glycol (anti-freeze), disease-causing animal viruses, formaldehyde, chlorinated hydrocarbons, and polysorbate 80, all of which are known carcinogens? There are also the food additives, MSG and aspartame, both of which are known to cause toxic, even fatal, allergic reactions. This fails to include the various animal protein components, which readily cause reactions, immune depression, and allergic shock. Reactions to foreign proteins may even cause sudden death.

Sudden infant death syndrome (SIDS) is almost assuredly due to vaccine-induced shock. The infant immune system is overwhelmed by the burdens of the vaccines—toxic animal proteins, harsh/toxic chemicals, mercury, food additives, and live or dead germs. The body systems go into shock, and the infant readily dies. Any infant who dies of sudden shock or so-called crib death within days, weeks, or months after a round of vaccinations, as well as so-called shaken baby syndrome, must be considered a vaccine victim until proven otherwise.

Cournoyer lists the chemicals most commonly found in vaccines as follows:

- synthetic phenol (made from coal tar), a deadly poison
- thimerasol, a highly toxic form of mercury formerly known as mercurochrome (or merthiolate)
- formaldehyde (also known as formalin)
- alum (a kind of aluminum salt used as a preservative) — it causes blood to coagulate
- aluminum phosphate (the same type of aluminum used in deodorants)
- acetone (a toxic solvent used in fingernail polish remover)

Other ingredients which may be found in vaccines include gelatin, residues of antibiotics, particularly neomycin, streptomycin, tetracycline, gentamycin, polymyxcin B sulfate, gelatin, sugar, yeast particles, and MSG. Due to the use of antibiotics the vaccines are contaminated by mold. Some vaccines may contain soy protein derivatives from genetically engineered soy. All such substances can elicit allergic reactions which can lead to potentially severe consequences, including shock and sudden death. In particular, reactions to soy may be severe, especially the genetically engineered variety. A person may be allergic to several of the ingredients in the vaccine, for instance, yeast, MSG, mold residues, and soy protein. When these are injected in the form of the vaccine serum in the sensitive adult, child, or infant there is a high risk of a reaction. The immune system and organs may react violently, resulting in shock, even death. This happens to thousands of people yearly. On a lesser scale there may be fever, aches, rash, chills, and fatigue. Or, at the minimum the consequences are immune suppression, which ultimately leads to chronic disease.

There is another factor regarding vaccine toxicity that is rarely considered. Millions of individuals are allergic to antibiotics. The majority of these drugs are derived from molds. What's more, the number of people who are reactive to molds is vast. Furthermore, there is no disclaimer on the injection to warn of these ingredients nor any package insert to forewarn. Thus, a person who is highly sensitive to antibiotics could react violently to the injection. Such reactions could include allergic shock, even sudden death. Thus, like synthetic food additives and antibiotics, vaccines are a major cause of sudden allergy-induced shock and death. What's more, the deaths are rarely recorded as vaccine-induced.

It is the standard of care that if a person is sensitive to antibiotics, his/her medical chart is flagged for that sensitivity. This is to protect that individual from sudden or life-threatening reactions. Such a person may even wear a protective bracelet warning medical authorities of the risk. The same should occur with vaccinations, that is there must be a warning to protect anyone who is allergic to antibiotics, even mold. No such person should take vaccines.

Vaccinations have destructive effects upon the immune system. They introduce a wide range of protein molecules, which greatly disrupt physiology. Such proteins are potent poisons capable of disabling virtually any organ. They contaminate the body with various residues of germ protein, as well as germ genetic material, which further burden it. They flood the bloodstream with serum and blood proteins from a wide range of animals and in some cases even from humans. What's more, they introduce a vast range of actual germs—bacteria, bacteria-like organisms, mycoplasmas, cell wall-deficients, fungi, yeasts, viruses, and virus-like particles. Some of these germs are alive, some dead, and some partially alive, or inactivated. Some are chemically altered but still functional, although they have been converted into a kind of microbial freak—the result of the treatment with harsh chemicals. Others are true aberrations of nature, genetically engineered mutants. Still others as a result of being exposed to radiation develop into bizarre forms, which are also elusive. These mutants often contain no cell wall, which makes them virtually unrecognizable. This means the immune system is unable to purge them. Thus, the germs gain residence within the cells and organs, where they cause chronic infections. Such germs are stealth invaders, and without resistance they invade the cells, causing a host of syndromes and diseases.

Vaccines contain a variety of germs. These germs greatly damage the immune system. There is great danger in the fact that vaccines contain mutated genes. These genes are often genetically altered to create super mutants, the freaks of nature. The reason for the danger is that the immune system is incapable of recognizing them. The ability of the immune system to destroy germs is based upon a surveillance system. What's more, this system is based upon detecting the cell wall: the body is able to recognize the existence of the germ based upon the proteins and components of the cell wall. So, the cell wall serves as a signal of the germ's presence. The cell walls of germs are disrupted or destroyed by harsh chemicals such as formaldehyde and mercurial compounds. However, many such germs continue to live in a mutated form. Thus, even though they are supposedly weakened they can still wreak havoc within the body. Once the cell wall is stripped from the germ the immune system has no way to recognize it. Thus, it invades the body uncontested.

There are three main types of stealth invaders: chemically inactivated germs, which largely lack cell walls or have disrupted cell walls, genetically engineered germs, which are foreign to nature, and antibiotic-resistant germs, which also have defective or disrupted cell walls secondary to the effects of these drugs. All such germs place a great burden upon the immune system and suppress it. There is yet another category: naturally occurring cell wall-deficient organisms, such as SV40 and various mycoplasmas, which may contaminate the vaccine solution.

There are potentially hundreds of such germs in vaccines. The fact is through vaccines individuals are contaminated with a vast array of germs that, incredibly, even the vaccine makers are unaware of. Thus, by infecting humans with such an enormous range of potentially destructive germs vaccines render the immune system incompetent. This is why people who are heavily vaccinated fail to mount an immune response. They suffer in a state of immune chronic depression. In other words, the immune systems of such persons are so burdened with vaccine-related germs and various injected toxins, such as thimerasol and formaldehyde, that there is little or no capacity for an active response. Thus, anyone who receives modern vaccines assumes a body burden of a wide range of toxins as well as cancer-causing germs.

Such individuals rarely develop the expected natural reaction to germs: fever, chills, aches, and malaise. Rather, they suffer from chronic maladies that largely evade diagnosis and for which, seemingly, no cause or cure can be found. They endure with a host of symptoms that devastate their lives and which appear inflammatory and/or infectious in nature, without the obvious symptoms so typical in acute infections. These are the individuals who are labeled with vague diagnoses: immune suppression, weak immune system, immune deficiency, fibromyalgia, chronic fatigue syndrome, polymyositis, viral syndrome, rheumatism, arthritis, chronic back pain, ankylosing spondylitis, and similar 'cause unknown' syndromes.

The governments claim to have the right to mandate vaccination policies. This is despite the fact that government has no 'license' to practice medicine. In 2004 the United States government 'required' that all infants and toddlers age 6 through 23 months must be vaccinated for the flu. Yet, was this truly an altruistic government mandate or was it merely a lust for money motivated by the desires of the drug cartel? Surely, no evidence for safety was presented, nor was there any proof of effectiveness. It was merely suddenly mandated. This is despite the fact that in other parts of the world, for instance, Japan, the giving of vaccines to children under five years is banned. This is also despite the content of mercury in the form of thimerasol, a known cause of brain damage. The EPA, FDA, and the American Academy of Pediatrics have all demanded the elimination of mercury from childhood vaccines. Yet, no ban has been enacted, and vaccines still contain this dangerous metal some five years after the EPA dictate.

The toxicity of mercury to the human brain is beyond dispute. Thousands of research studies document its deadly effects. A recent study fully confirmed the monumental danger of this substance. In June 2004, Dr. Mady Hornig of Columbia

University released the results of her incriminating findings: mercury in the same levels as found in common childhood vaccines damages the developing brain. Dr. Hornig concluded that this leads to behavioral and neurological damage. The government itself has confirmed these findings, since Congress has held investigations detailing the tainted relationship between government offices and vaccine makers. The fact is rather than proven science it is mere pharmaceutical lobbying which leads to vaccine mandates.

It was Special Counsel to Congress, Scott J. Bloch, who said that the evidence, that is the science, behind vaccines is "inconclusive." What's more, said Bloch, the toxicity and potential harm of mercury in human vaccines must be reevaluated, since this metal is a "potent neurotoxin." Thus, even key government offices are aware of the poisonous nature of this compound, fully cognizant that the vaccines are poisoning humans.

Again, vaccines are not mandated by medical authorities. Rather, they are mandated by the government. Says Special Counsel Bloch, "the vaccine program is administered by the U.S. Department of Health and Human Services. In his letters to Congress the Special Counsel makes every effort to awaken the government to this danger, stating, in his letter to the U.S. Senate dated May 20, 2004, that the evidence is clear that there is a "substantial and specific danger to public health caused by the use of thimerasol/mercury in vaccines." This, he claims, is due to the "inherent toxicity" of mercurial compounds. Such a toxicity was known by the government, while any such danger was ignored. Worse, a coverup is alleged. Says Bloch:

> ...the CDC and the Food and Drug Administration colluded with pharmaceutical companies at a conference in Norcross, Georgia, in June 2000, to prevent the release of a study which showed a statistical correlation between thimerasol/mercury

exposure through pediatric vaccines and neurological disorders, including autism, Attention-Deficit/ Hyperactivity Disorder, stuttering, tics, and speech and language delays. Instead of releasing the data presented at the conference, the author of the study, Dr. Thomas Verstaeten, later published a different version of the study in the November 2003 issue of Pediatrics, which did not show a statistical correlation. No explanation has been provided for this discrepancy. Finally, the disclosures allege that there is an increasing body of clinical evidence on the connection of thimerasol/mercury exposure to neurological disorders which is being ignored by government...agencies.

Yet, even though the aforementioned words are powerful on the government level no action was taken. This proved to be merely a protest from Bloch, since his organization has no power to enforce its findings. The fact is his findings were routinely ignored by government officials, who even attempted to refute them. This is despite the fact that one of the world's top neurologists, Baylor College's Dr. David Baskin, at Congressional hearings proclaimed that at a minimum there was "no reason to continue to *purposely inject* (mercury) into the bloodstream of infants."

The vaccines given to infants, toddlers, and children contain mercury at levels up to 12.5 micrograms per injection. This is sufficient to cause potentially permanent brain damage. Surely, it is enough to cause behavioral disorders, even retardation. This is only a portion of this catastrophe. Says Russell L. Blaylock, M.D., one of the world's leading neurosurgeons, "aluminum (is) found in all childhood vaccines", which is a cause of "neurodegenerative diseases such as Alzheimer's dementia, ALS (Lou Gehrig's disease), and Parkinson's disease." The fact is Blaylock is opposed to the systematic vaccination of children, particularly infants, with any mercury- or aluminum-laced vaccines. Regarding this supposed therapy he says, "To start children at age 6 months receiving yearly doses of aluminum and mercury is insane. To subject...children to this danger, given the fact that in over 50% of the cases the wrong virus is used to make the vaccine, makes the recommendation even more absurd. The (medical profession) has shown itself to be irresponsible..." Then, Blaylock bravely proclaims, "Mothers should be warned to avoid flu vaccines for their children and themselves. Instead, they should be advised to breast-feed their babies, take (the appropriate supplements during pregnancy and nursing), and provide multi-vitamins added to a good diet for their children."

According to the VRAN (Vaccine Risk Awareness Network), a non-profit organization, there is a degree of conspiracy with these injections. The organization claims that vaccines are promoted through "propaganda", which is barraged at parents, urging them to vaccinate "all healthy children and babies starting at age 6 months." As evidence they quote Canadian physician Dr. Sherry Tenpenny, who exposed the vaccine propaganda machine by writing about the conference, "The Seven-Step Recipe for Generating Interest in, and Demand for, Flu Vaccination." This exposé is described on the Web site vran.org. The organization in particular attempts to educate Canadian citizens, who are heavily targeted with such propaganda. Say the authors:

> Your babies and children are the new target market for this (flu) vaccine experiment. Recently, a news segment on CBC's The National implanted the idea that it is children who spread the flu to others, and, therefore, vaccinating babies and young children prevents its spread...The Canadian media is dutifully pumping out flu vaccine propaganda without pausing to inquire what negative heath impact this may have on

children's health in the short or long term, nor how one would determine a 6 month old baby's sensitivity to vaccine ingredients like egg, thimerasol, neomycin (an antibiotic). And no one is reporting a recent study which shows a poor immune response in infants to influenza vaccination.

SV40: Western pandemic

Evidence exists that childhood diabetes is a direct result of vaccinations—the SV40 appears to be a cofactor in this as well. Thus, vaccine viruses and toxins are responsible for a certain number of childhood deaths from diabetes or its complications. It is truly beyond comprehension how any 'authorities' could regard the use of animal tissues/blood, including monkey tissue, as a safe medium. Regarding the use of monkeys, usually, the kidneys are utilized. Regarding human tissue placenta is the source. With dogs it is also kidney tissue. All such organs carry disease-causing germs.

The use of monkey kidney and testicular tissue is particularly bizarre. These are excretory organs, and, thus, they are rife with contamination. Plus, due to their intimate relationship with the genitals, surely, they house potentially sexually transmitted germs. No sensible person would use such tissues for creating medicines for humans.

The process for making the vaccine is telling. The actual monkey kidneys and genitals were ground up and used in the growth media. Surely, no one with even the slightest common sense would expect that such tissue was a safe source. Surely, financial interests superceded human concerns.

It is catastrophic to create a medicine based upon a "mad rush" or "competing egos." Yet, regarding the Sabin and Salk vaccines this was what occurred: who could get to market first with the product that earned the largest government contract.

Safety and deliberate science were never a consideration. For those who are skeptical of this claim the fact is safety was purposely overlooked. For instance, regarding the Sabin vaccine, the oral sugar cube was soaked in vaccine solution. This was a solution containing known contaminants, namely the SV40 virus. Incredibly, government officials were well aware of the potential harm from the vaccine but administered it regardless.

The government had already promoted its value. It was 'embarrassed' at the thought of such a revelation, that is that the vaccine was poisonous. Incredibly, in 1960 before it was launched it was discovered that it was contaminated: with SV40 among other agents. The launch date was 1962 to 1963. The government decided to go forward, 'despite unknown risks—despite the known contamination with a cancer-causing virus.' Government officials claimed if the contamination was revealed, "people might lose trust in government policies." Apparently, this was the primary reason that the vaccine was forced through—again, despite concerns of researchers of long-term damage. The researchers were ignored: government policy superceded them. As a result, millions have been sickened, many with 'incurable' cancers as well as a vast array of neurological disorders.

As a result of this misguided policy, which lacked any sound or scientific basis and, rather, violated the available science, tens of thousands, perhaps millions, have died a most brutal death: from brain, lung, blood, muscle, and bone cancers. To confirm this all that needs to be done is to study the MD Anderson Web site, as well as the work of Michelle Carbone, M.D., which proves that, in fact, deadly cancers are directly due to simian virus 40. Again, rather than a truly wild or animal virus this is a man-created virus injected into humans by the hands of their fellow humans. There is an SV40 in monkeys, but it is different than the one which is epidemic in humans.

Humans create their own catastrophes. Then, amazingly, they blame God for their miseries, when the real cause is the faulty thinking of humankind—this faulty greedy thinking and deliberate vile acts—which cause harm to others. The holy books teach that the individual must live by a special law, that is the Golden Rule—to treat others as the individual himself would want to be treated.

What a fantastic rule it is! If people lived by it, this Earth would be a paradise. Consider the words of the Qur'an, that is that if a person saves the life of a single individual it is as if he/she saved the life of the entire human race, but if a single person is wrongly killed, it is as if the perpetrator has destroyed all of humanity: these are words to give deep consideration. The point is that because of the sugar cube and injectable polio vaccines, innocent people have died. They number in the tens of thousands. Almighty God tells the human beings to above all avoid causing each other harm. The fact is this is the teaching of the sages of the past. This is the only way of thinking which can save the human race.

If the human race is to survive, the philosophy of modern civilization must change. Merely creating a product only for financial benefit—only for the benefit of reputation, fame, and power—while neglecting to consider higher needs, this is the cause of civilization's doom. This was precisely the case with the polio vaccine. During its inception numerous scientists issued warnings that the systematic injection or intake of this vaccine would lead to human harm. This is precisely what occurred. This explains the title of the British researcher M. Beddow Bayly's monograph, *The Salk Vaccine Disaster*. This was the conclusion of British investigators a mere year after the vaccine was launched, and it was based upon the symptoms and side effects, as well as the deaths, directly attributed to it. Bayly was well aware of the contamination issues. Perhaps this was why the vaccine was so brazenly rushed to market before scientists fully publicized its dangers—before the truth about it was fully revealed.

To these early researchers the conspiratorial nature of the push for the vaccine was readily apparent. He notes that it was well published in *The Lancet* that during the era of the vaccination call "there (was)...a...definite risk that the vaccine may produce (paralysis). Obviously, for British researchers this was a definite concern, which caused some investigators to veto mass vaccination. One researcher, Dr. Geffen, then noted that "It is not easy to be sure that in all batches of vaccine produced on a commercial scale the virus will be dead, and in trials of a vaccine some years ago in America some 12 children did develop poliomyelitis after injection, paralysis affecting chiefly the limb of injection or the contralateral limb." What's more, incredibly, these researchers noted that the more of such vaccines an individual received—recall that the injectable Salk vaccine called for several additional booster shots—the greater is the risk for damage. For instance, as "categorically stated" in *The Lancet* three injections increased the risks for infection of the central nervous system three-fold.

Albert Sabin, M.D., the inventor of the oral polio vaccine, condemned the injectable type as "dangerous." Incredibly, in 1955 this physician testified before a House of Representative Subcommittee about its danger, yet, within a few years launched his own largely unproven polio vaccine. It was then well known by Sabin and others that the injectable vaccine led to shedding, meaning that the vaccinated person acted as a carrier, causing the outbreak of the disease in susceptible individuals. In other words, the vaccine itself caused outbreaks of polio not only in the vaccinated, but also in the people who fail to get vaccinated.

Could any improvement be expected from Sabin's vaccine, which contained live viruses? Incredibly, during his appearance before the House Subcommittee Sabin's purpose was never for humanitarian issues. It was merely to popularize his own contrary agenda—his own oral vaccine. The fact is it was the oral vaccine which proved even more deadly than the injectable one. This is because it created a far broader epidemic than outbreaks of polio: the modern cancer epidemic.

There is also danger, said these early researchers, in the injection of monkey kidney tissue, which inevitably contaminates the vaccine. As reported in the *Manchester Guardian* one of Britain's greatest researchers documented that the frequent or repeated inoculation of vaccines derived from monkey organs is "terrifying in its possibilities." One of his concerns was the inevitable occurrence of anaphylactic shock, which could lead to sudden death. In fact, with modern vaccines this is a relatively common although underreported, complication. Various toxic allergic reactions, this researcher proposed, were likely. What's more, reported the *Guardian,* "there is a risk, of unknown dimensions, that repeated injection of a vaccine prepared from monkey kidney may eventually sensitize the child in some harmful way." Incredibly, the *Guardian* quoted researchers, who admitted that there was no scientific basis for the vaccine. Much was based upon speculation. Say the researchers:

> We do not know how long immunity it confers or whether booster shots are required...There was also the possibility that immunization of young children might transfer the danger of polio infection to a later group, those, say, between 18 and 35, when the contraction of the disease is much more serious and far more difficult to cure.

Incredibly, this is precisely what occurred in a boarding school on the East Coast, when nearly 180 students contracted polio. All students contracted it within the school. Half the victims were people who failed to get vaccinated, while the other half were probably (vaccinated) carriers. The most likely scenario was that a vaccinated carrier transmitted the disease to the people who failed to get vaccinated.

Chemicals or viruses: which is the culprit?

Surely, this epidemic was due to the vaccine virus, that is hidden viruses, which escape the supposed 'sterilization.' What's more, the sterilization agents themselves are largely responsible. Both formaldehyde and mercury are potent neurotoxins, capable of causing brain damage. Plus, such substances alter the structure of the blood-brain barrier, increasing the risks for brain infections such as polio.

Drug companies claim that mercury, as injected in vaccines, is relatively safe. Government offices join this with claims of low or no mercury content in modern vaccines. Regarding the claim by some Canadian authorities that the vaccine no longer contains mercury says the VRAN Web site:

> Pharmaceutical giants Aventis Pasteur and ID Biomedical are the...main flu vaccine suppliers in Canada. The contents of Aventis Pasteur's vaccine Vaxigrip still contain thimerasol in multivial doses. Babies and young children are injected with half the standard dose twice, each dose 4 weeks apart, and will presumably receive vaccine drawn from a multidose vials containing the mercury based preservative. The vaccine also contains formaldehyde...Biomedical's vaccine (is known as) Fluviral.

What's more, Aventis Pasteur's own monograph cautions "this vaccine should not be administered to anyone with a history of hypersensitivity and especially anaphylactic reactions to eggs or egg products. It is also a contraindication to administer this vaccine to individuals known to be sensitive to thimerasol...or neomycin." Regarding antibiotics, such as neomycin, hundreds of thousands of American and Canadian children are reactive. Incredibly, some one in five infants and children are egg-sensitive. What's more, virtually all infants and children react negatively to exposure to mercury. Thus, can any infant or child safely take such vaccines?

Regarding the bizarre nature of the government's vaccination project the VRAN Web site provides additional revealing data. Quoting the Health Canada Web site:

> Three influenza vaccines are licensed for use in Canada...All three are sterile suspensions prepared from influenza viruses propagated in chicken embryos. The virus is inactivated, purified and treated with an organic solvent to remove surface glycoproteins, producing a "split-virus" preparation that is intended to reduce vaccine reactogenicity. One dose...of vaccine contains...three antigens. The antigens chose for inclusion in influenza vaccine are reviewed annually to ensure that they include antigens that are expected to provided the best protection during the following winter. All three licensed vaccines use thimerasol (0.01%) as preservative. Gelatin (0.05%) is used as a stabilizer...

Note the second sentence in the aforementioned quote: *sterile suspensions*. No one offers any proof for sterility. Health Canada takes the drug company literature at face value. They do no testing, offering no confirmation of such sterility, which is critical.

In their toxicity vaccinations are systemic. The injection of even a single germ can lead to systemic disease. Recall that it was once claimed that the 1950s- and 1960s- era polio injection was sterile, yet, hundreds of North Americans developed polio from it. Now, are people to believe mere company literature, that is without any proof or documentation?

There is additional evidence for a lack of sterility. Note that the growth medium is living cells, that is the cells of chicken embryos. This means that the vaccine contains potentially a wide range of viruses, as well as other germs, such as mycoplasmas, bacteria, and parasites, which infect chickens.

No screening is done to ensure that these viruses and germs are not introduced into the vaccines. What's more, these are commercial eggs, which are used for the propagation. This means that through such a production various mad cow-like agents could be introduced. This is because commercial chickens are fed chow derived from rendered animals products, the source of the mad cow epidemic. According to Richard Rhodes in his book, *Deadly Feasts*, the introduction of mad cow-like agents directly into the bloodstream, which is achieved by modern vaccinations, increases the risks for the development of this syndrome a million-fold, that is as compared to the oral route.

There is also the issue of the use of organic solvents in such vaccines. Such solvents, made from petroleum residues, are potent carcinogens. They are condemned for human consumption due to the heightened risk for liver damage and death. Yet, they are freely injected in humans, even babies, without restriction.

This is criminal, to put people at risk, merely for corporate profits. Yet, the true debacle is that there is no guarantee for sterility: for instance, SV40, which is a likely contaminant in chicken embryo-based vaccines, is resistant to such solvents, including formaldehyde. What's more, hundreds of other infectious agents are resistant to such solvents. Thus, there is no proof that the common flu shot is sterile. The claim that it contains only dead germs is implausible. What's more, tens of thousands of individuals have developed bizarre sicknesses from flu shots, and these sicknesses fully appear as infectious in nature. Yet, in what is an even more profound revelation of the defective nature of the vaccination program the Health Canada dissertation notes that the vaccine is "expected" to be corrected, that is there is no true scientific basis for it. Rather, it is based upon guesswork.

Is it worth risking an individual's life, in fact, the lives of millions of people, including babies, based upon a supposedly educated guess? The fact is there is no scientific basis for the modern flu vaccine. What's more, there is no mention of what is the source of the influenza virus, which is grown, harvested, and, then, injected into humans. Is it monkey virus, rodent virus, chicken virus, or human virus? Is it a perhaps from pigs? If it is from pigs, since these animals are similar genetically to humans, could the porcine virus genes delve into the human genes, creating a mutant?

Could such a mutant, then, just as had occurred in chicken embryos, refurbish itself in humans, creating a pig-human hybrid, a true freak of nature capable of devastating the human race? No such production can be ruled out, in fact, such a scenario is inevitable. Vaccine viruses contains vital materials, including the genes of influenza viruses, which could readily splice with human cells.

The vaccine companies need to report the source of the viruses. If it is from pigs, as was the case with the original Swine Flu vaccine, no one should be inoculated due to the risk of the creation of an epidemic. This happened in 1918, since the source of the killer flu epidemic was, incredibly, vaccinated soldiers. Today, the same scenario is likely, since there is a war and since the soldiers are extensively vaccinated—who are regularly re-entering the United States and who, then, could be the progenitors of the next pandemic. Plus, procine viruses are notoriously associated with cancer. Thus, every time such viruses are injected the cancer risks accelerate. The value of the divine prohibition against pork becomes evident. What's more, people claim there is no God.

Yet, the drug companies ignore the divine law. The VRAN Web site provides further information regarding this debacle. What follows is the contents of the package insert for the flu vaccine Vaxigrip by Aventis Pasteur:

> *VAXIGRIP...Inactivated Influenza Vaccine Trivalent Types A and B...for intramuscular use, is a sterile suspension prepared from influenza viruses propagated in chicken embryos. The virus-containing fluids are harvested and the virus inactivated with formaldehyde and purified by zonal centrifugation. The virus is then chemically disrupted using (an ethylene glycol-like substance, a type of anti-freeze), producing a "split-antigen". The split antigen is suspended in sodium phosphate-buffered, isotonic sodium chloride solution.*

Then, for instance, for the year 2002 to 2003 vaccine key ingredients are listed, for instance:

• the A-Panama virus or its residues
• the A-New Calendonia virus or its residues
• the B-Shangdong (that is B-Hong Kong) virus or its residues
• thimerasol (mercury)
• formaldehyde
• ethylene glycol
• sugar
• neomycin

All such substances are toxic. Many cause acute and potentially fatal allergic reactions, including allergic shock, heart arrhythmia, and sudden death, that is from cardiac standstill. The aforementioned chemicals are a primary cause of toxicity, tissue damage, organ disruption, and disease.

There is another serious question which is never addressed. This is the issue of the origin of the viruses—that is the ones used to make the vaccines—for instance, the viruses mentioned in the aforementioned vaccines, the A-Panama, the A-New Caledonia, and the B-Shangdong. According to the WHO these are largely derived from pigs, swabbed from their snouts and, then, cultured in chicken eggs.

Naturally, this porcine virus would interact with the genetic material from chickens. This would lead to a combination virus, part chicken and part pig. Then, when such a virus—or the viral genetic material derived from them—is injected into humans, it could become part porcine, ovine (bird), and human. This is deadly. This would be a catastrophe wrought by modern medicine with its unscientific, in fact, barbaric approach—its methods devoid of scientific basis, its techniques based upon mere "guesswork," in fact, mere arrogance. People who are injected with such vaccines derived from pigs or poultry will surely become ill: in a epidemic many will die.

There is no scientific basis for modern vaccines. Yet, few people realize it.

On the contrary there is evidence only that the vaccines are poisonous. The evidence of this toxicity is so compelling that the legislature of certain states, especially California and Iowa, voted to ban certain vaccine ingredients, notably mercury. In California a bill was passed prohibiting doctors from injecting vaccines containing thimerasol. This is telling. Obviously, the legislatures were exposed to a plethora of evidence, proving the destructive nature of this substance.

Mercury is toxic to infants and pregnant women. It readily accumulates in the infantile brain as well as the fetal womb. It fully poisons the embryo's developing brain, causing destruction of neurons. This results in developmental delay, and, therefore, retardation. These are proven facts, yet, supposed authorities in the United States and Canada proclaim that it is "hard to pinpoint whether or not people are having adverse reactions" to this poison and, what's more, "the safety of the shots and the benefits far outweigh the risks." Yet, it was the University of Calgary's Faculty of Medicine which conducted studies on this metal's noxious effects upon humans, finding categorically that mercury causes "rapid damage to the nerve cells." This is true even in the minute amounts found in vaccines. Thus, in light of such research it is essentially criminal to suggest, let alone mandate, the injection of such a compound.

In foods the lacing of any item with mercury is prohibited. Why should it be allowed in medicines—these too are ingestible or 'injectable.' Rather, regarding vaccinations it would be even more critical to avoid such an intake, since there is no means for the body to protect itself against injected toxins. The toxins may enter directly into critical tissues, such as the brain, liver, and kidneys, where they can cause permanent damage. Thus, even rather minor amounts of such toxins can lead to extreme damage. This is particularly true of the direct injection of mercury, which is readily absorbed into the brain. There it will aggressively cause brain cell damage.

Mercury binds to human proteins, causing them to be destroyed. It also readily absorbs into the fat—the brain is mostly fatty tissue. This metal's destructive actions are largely due to its effects upon enzymes, which it irreversibly destroys. Thus, it should never be added to a 'medicine': nor should it ever be injected into the human body. The injection of mercury into the human body has never been proven safe. Thus, all such injections should be halted immediately. In other words, the injection of mercury-laced vaccines should be immediately banned.

Yet, the medical profession continues to promote the use of such vaccines, while lacking any proof of safety. In contrast, a plethora of research documents the dire consequences of injectable mercury. Incredibly, despite repeated warnings, even by federal agencies, regarding the danger of this substance the CDC continues to recommend it. According to its guidelines various supposedly high risk individuals must get the flu vaccine, including "pregnant women in the second or third trimester", even going so far to claim that "there is no evidence that flu vaccine administered during the first trimester of pregnancy is harmful to the fetus or mother." These are utter lies. It is despite the categorical evidence by hundreds of independent investigators that, in fact, the components of this vaccine are highly destructive to the developing brain. Mercury causes brain damage, yet, "medical authorities," such as the Mayo Clinic and the CDC, both of which are heavily vested with the drug cartel, continue to recommend it, insisting it is safe. This demonstrates the hypocrisy of the medical profession, whose oath would appear to be "above all protect the monopoly first."

The public trusts such sources. Yet, these sources fail to tell the truth, rather, they freely lie. This is in order to maintain the status quo, even though there is no evidence for their position. The injection of mercury-containing vaccines causes disease. Those who deem it safe have their own vested positions. The fact is the Mayo Clinic and the CDC are funded by the drug companies. They are financially indebted to such companies. This is why despite evidence of human toxicity they continue to promote this agenda.

The CDC makes the guidelines. The major medical institutions 'religiously' follow them. Both the CDC and the great medical institutions of this country are dependent upon drug company funding. Then, is it possible to trust the medical mandates from such sources?

The system is corrupt. Thus, the dictates arising from the system must also be corrupt. Regarding vaccine mandates no such recommendations can be trusted. The fact is such recommendations are based upon financial concerns rather than significant science.

There is no science proving that the flu vaccine is either safe or effective. Thus, why take it?

The government aggressively promotes the vaccine agenda. Vast amounts of taxpayer money are expended in such promotions. Essentially, the government is in the vaccine business, although the payee is the common taxpayer. Yet, those in government positions who are responsible for mandating this approach are often not medically trained. Does it make sense to accept dictates from people who lack any medical education? Why follow a program that is based upon a government agenda rather than the summation of the science? Until there is proof that the vaccine is both safe and effective it makes sense to avoid taking it. The fact is the Mayo Clinic and the CDC are in the drug-promotion business. Regarding the use of various drugs and vaccines they cannot be trusted, because their position is compromised. Do not take the CDC and Mayo Clinic recommendations as gospel. They lack independence. It is the CDC and Mayo Clinic among dozens of other orthodox medical organizations which brazenly recommended flu shots for infants.

Curt Andersen, in his article from the *Green Bay News-Chronical*, documents the dire nature of this fallacy. He reminds us that the tolerance of tiny humans for this poison is low. Because of their developmental state they are highly vulnerable to neurotoxins. This is common knowledge, well established in the medical literature. Yet, he says, mothers of potentially vaccine-damaged children have recently discovered a cover-up: that there is "selective use (by the government and drug companies) of data to eliminate the associations in earlier studies between autism and vaccines containing mercury."

According to Andersen during the 1990s the government 'mandated' that to enter school children had to undergo an increase in vaccinations. However, the government failed to adhere to its own guidelines for childhood exposure to mercury. Then, tiny "two-month old babies were getting up to 62.5 micrograms of mercury, nearly 118 times the EPA's limit for daily exposure *for an adult*. Tests of baby teeth have shown very high levels of mercury after inoculations at that age." The high levels of mercury in the babies' teeth is clear evidence of vaccine-induced poisoning. There could be no other legitimate source for such poisoning. What's more, the measurement of such levels is categorical evidence for the contamination of the infants' brains with this metal. This means that, surely, there will be developmental delay or some similar consequences for any infant so extensively contaminated.

It is easy to prove that the government isn't really a government. Rather, it is a business operated by relatively few people who are protecting vested interests. Consider the so-called Homeland Security Act, the massive bill which arose after the 9/11 catastrophe. According to Bob Herbert, columnist for the *New York Times*, "Buried in this massive bill, covertly placed into it in the dark of the night by persons unknown was a provision that, incredibly, will protect Eli Lilly and other big pharmaceutical outfits from lawsuits by parents who believe their children were harmed by thimerasol."

Later, the true culprits were discovered: high authorities from the White House itself instructed the House Majority Leader, Dick Arney, to insert it. When confronted, Mr. Arney bragged about it, saying he was proud of it, the secretive insertion, in other words, he was rebellious. Surely, financially, Mr. Arney is connected to such concerns. It was Senator John McCain of Arizona who stated the obvious, that the insertion of such language "will primarily benefit large brand-name pharmaceutical companies, which produce additives to children's vaccines...It has no bearing whatsoever on domestic security." In contrast, Arney said that the White House instructed him to insert the language at the last minute to avoid debate.

Eli Lilly, in fact, makes mercurial compounds. They are largely the originators of mercury-based antiseptics such as mercurochrome and merthiolate (that is thimerasol). This company has an exceedingly close relationship with the Bush family. George Bush, Sr., served on the board of this company. During recent presidencies, including the various Bush presidencies, numerous White House officials have served as Lilly officials. Incredibly, in what is raw evidence of the corrupt nature of the relationship Sidney Taurel, the CEO of Eli Lilly, serves on the President's Homeland Security Advisory Counsel. Thus, obviously, the drug companies routinely buy favors. Taurel had effectively made it a terrorist act to criticize his company. As further evidence of the tainted nature of the relationship Andersen notes:

> ...numerous legislators own millions of dollars' worth of stocks in drug companies...just in case you were wondering why you are still paying (high prices) for prescription medicine and why over 44% of American people are uninsured while untold millions are one step away from being uninsured. There are no ethics rules or laws that prohibit stock ownership by legislators. What would ordinarily be considered conflict of interest in any jerkwater town is A-OK for Washington fat-cats.

He continued:

> ...concerns about elevated mercury levels have led the EPA and FDA to issue warnings to vulnerable populations, such as pregnant women and small

children, to limit consumption of fish, especially from the Great Lakes. This past December, EPA recommended that emissions from...power plants be dramatically reduced...Most industrial sources of mercury have been phased out in the United States, but...antibiotic tinctures like Mercurochrome and Merthiolate, dental amalgam...

This brings up a key point: in schools it is now banned in chemistry class to experiment with mercury. The old 'playing with a ball of mercury' is illegal. Even in the making of thermometers, due to its high degree of toxicity both to workers and those who accidentally are exposed to the residues, it is banned. So, how could it be allowed to be routinely injected into babies? This is a fraud of the highest degree.

The scope of this fraud has been recently confirmed by a Columbia University study. There, investigators determined that the administration of mercury in tiny amounts, such as the amounts found in childhood vaccines, causes brain damage, especially in the developing brain. According to Dr. Mady Hornig "the connection" between mercury and brain damage has been clearly identified, while the only solution is to limit or eliminate childhood exposure.

As demonstrated by the Columbia University study the CDC's position that mercury in vaccines is non-toxic is fraudulent. It is a kind of government 'spin': an attempt to protect big-money interests. There is no scientific basis for claiming a lack of evidence against mercury. Clearly, this substance, particularly when injected into the developing infant, is poisonous.

Investigators in Britain are also pointing to the toxic actions of this substance. According to Rosie Waterhouse of the *UK Times,* "Mercury in vaccines for babies and infants could be the cause of a steep rise in cases of autism in children...according to a growing number of scientists." The increase in autism in

Britain and the United States, she reports, is directly associated with the increase in the number of inoculations given to young children. Thimerasol itself, she notes, is nearly 50% mercury by weight, a substance with proven brain-damaging actions.

Autism is a disorder represented by symptoms of brain damage in children, which may include inability to communicate, learning impairment, retardation, and bizarre violent behavior. Incredibly, notes Waterhouse, the symptoms of mercury poisoning in children are similar to those found in autism. She also reports that in the Western world from 1984 to 1994 the incidence of autism has risen some tenfold. This coincides precisely with the increase in the use of mercury-contaminated vaccines. Thus, she quotes Boyd Haley, professor of chemistry at the University of Kentucky, who reported in a detailed scientific analysis that "Thimerasol is extremely toxic" and that "vaccines are the most likely suspect for causing autism." The fact is in the United States there has been a vast increase in this disease, and, what's more, it coincides directly with the increase in vaccination. Need anything further be said—the fact is mercury-containing vaccines must be banned immediately. Furthermore, she reports:

> ...the cumulative effects of mercury impair brain development and damage the child's immune system and gastrointestinal tract, resulting in hypersensitivity to toxic environmental substances. Thus, build-up could lead to autism or a form of mercury poisoning...In addition, researchers believe, the MMR triple vaccine, usually given at 18 months to two years, could trigger autism because the damaged immune system cannot cope with three live viruses at once.

This demonstrates that autism could be a combination of immune or brain damage from the toxic compounds in the vaccines as well as vaccine-induced viral infections. There is no proof that vaccines are entirely germ free. Surely, a certain number of germs or potentially biologically active germ DNA enter the body through these injections. Surely, these agents cause human disease. What's more, mercury damages the blood-brain barrier, increasing the ease of invasion by such germs or germ DNA into the brain. This may largely explain the rapid decline of children's health after vaccinations.

The degree of damage caused by vaccinations is beyond comprehension. Untold millions of children are poisoned by them. The flu vaccine mandated for children is poisonous, as are the standard childhood vaccines such as the MMR and DPT. Waterhouse notes that in a single multidose protocol, the equivalent of two shots, an infant/child will receive some 62.5 micrograms of thimerasol, a criminally high amount—certainly enough to cause brain damage. The fact is, says Waterhouse, this is some 100 times more than the EPA's proposed supposedly safe intake for a six-month-old.

The CDC itself has determined that the vaccines are causing harm and has largely attributed it to the mercury content. However, now, due to fears of legal redress, the CDC and the federal government are engaged in a massive cover-up. The objective is to convince the general public that the mercury in vaccines is relatively safe and that there is no evidence of harm. This is to minimize their liability for supporting the use of this destructive method. The fact is the CDC and the FDA alone are liable for criminal acts, since their enforced vaccine policy has caused numerous mercury-related diseases, including attention deficit, retardation, and autism.

Despite their claims for safety there is a plethora of independent research which proves precisely the opposite. This is confirmed by Tulane University's J. M. El-Dahr, prominent immunologist, who made it clear that all vaccines must be made "thimerasol-free." Yet, despite the dominating statements of such prominent scientists the governments of the United States and Europe have done virtually nothing to protect the public from these dangerous injections.

Metals in the brain: a vaccine syndrome?

The heavy metal content of vaccines is significant. It is significant enough to cause measurable heavy metal poisoning. The major metals found in vaccines are mercury and aluminum. Both are neurotoxic. Metals can be detected through blood testing or specialized testing of the hair and nails. Or, for a simpler method, which is equally as accurate as laboratory testing, a symptom analysis is useful. The fact is heavy metal poisoning creates predictable symptoms, and this is why a self-test is invaluable.

In June 1999, the FDA 'discovered' that "Infants who receive thimerasol-containing vaccines at several visits may have been exposed to more mercury than recommended by Federal guidelines." Within a month the European Agency of the Evaluation of Medical Products (EMEA) issued a statement saying, "Cumulative exposure to ethylmercury as found in thimerasol...could lead to (potential damage). Thus, the government is fully appraised of the dangerous nature of injectable mercury. This mercury accumulates in the brain and spinal cord, along with mercury from other sources, ultimately causing disease.

A detailed test for heavy metals has been provided. This test focuses primarily on the signs and symptoms of mercury poisoning. However, a high score may also indicate a generalized heavy metal intoxication. The focus is also on the symptoms commonly seen in recipients of multiple vaccines. Take this test to determine if you have mercury and/or heavy metal poisoning.

Add up the points to get your score.
Which of these applies to you?

Symptoms/Signs	Points/Value
1. numbness and tingling, especially in the tips of the fingers and the bottom of the feet	(4)
2. loss of sensation in the extremities	(3)
3. slow mental function	(2)
4. loss of control of the muscles	(3)
5. wasting of the muscles	(3)
6. metallic taste in mouth	(2)
7. tendency to develop yeast infections	(1)
8. yeast infections of the mouth or gums	(2)
9. epilepsy	(3)
10. spastic muscles	(2)
11. spastic spine	(2)
12. stiff spine	(2)
13. multiple sclerosis	(3)
14. ALS	(5)
15. tremors	(2)
16. retardation	(3)
17. seizures	(2)
18. muscular dystrophy	(3)
19. irritability	(1)
20. decline in mental function or intelligence	(1)
21. insomnia	(1)
22. memory loss	(1)
23. anxiety/nervousness	(1)
24. constant drowsiness	(1)

25. bleeding gums   (1)
26. coated tongue or oral thrush   (1)
27. excessive salivation   (3)
28. inflammation of the mouth or tongue   (1)
29. foul breath   (1)
30. abdominal cramps   (1)
31. vague stomach or intestinal problems   (1)
32. ringing in the ears   (1)
33. irregular heartbeat   (1)
34. feeble pulse   (1)
35. persistent chest pain or pressure   (1)
36. persistent headaches   (1)
37. dizziness   (1)
38. tremors of the eyelids or tongue   (3)
39. muscle weakness   (1)
40. fatigue   (1)
41. nerve deafness   (1)
42. low body temperature   (1)
43. excessive perspiration   (1)
44. shallow or irregular breathing   (1)
45. loss of appetite   (1)
46. weight loss   (1)
47. personality changes   (1)
48. psychotic tendencies   (1)
49. blue discoloration or lines in mouth   (3)
50. pain in extremities   (1)
51. depression and/or apathy   (1)
52. paralysis   (2)
53. difficulty speaking or garbled speech   (2)
54. unsteady gait   (3)
55. visual disorders   (1)
56. sudden or gradual hearing loss   (1)

57. chronic kidney disorder   (1)
58. Did you play with or touch a mercury ball
    (as a youngster, etc.)?   (3)
59. obvious silver or gray discoloration of the gums   (4)
60. Are you exposed to mercury
    (or other heavy metals) at work?   (3)
61. Do you have amalgam (silver) fillings in your mouth?
    • one to two fillings   (2)
    • three to five fillings   (3)
    • six to eight fillings   (5)
    • nine to ten fillings   (6)
    • eleven or more fillings   (8)
62. Are/were your amalgam fillings particularly large? (3)
63. Did you use to have such fillings but they
    have been replaced with non-metallic ones?   (2)
64. Do you have a combination of gold   (5)
    and silver (amalgam) fillings in your mouth?
65. Do you rarely eat red meat,   (4)
    eating instead mostly fish?
66. Do you eat swordfish, shark, or   (5)
    marlin a few times yearly?
67. Have you had the several traditional   (5)
    vaccines during your lifetime?

Answer only one of the following:

68. Do you eat ocean fish one or more times per week? (4)
69. Do you eat ocean fish three or more times per week? (6)

Your score _____

Evaluation of your score

2 to 10 points Possible/probable mercury intoxication:
Mercury has contaminated the entire globe. The levels of mercury in the atmosphere, water, and land are hundreds of times higher than they were 200 years ago. The industrial companies have effectively contaminated virtually every inch of the earth with this poison. Thus, all humans have a certain body burden of mercury.

The level of the mercury in the body determines the degree of the symptoms. So does body weight: a thin person is more likely to develop toxicity than a heavy person. Mercury is difficult to extract from the tissues. This is because it lodges deep within fatty tissues. Plus, it binds to cellular proteins. It poisons enzymes by adhering to them. Vitamin C is a major mercury antagonist, as is citric acid, that is the acid of tart fruit. So is tartaric acid, the acid of grapes and other sour fruit. This substance is found in large amounts in the red sour grape formula known as Resvital. To help cleanse heavy metals take one teaspoon daily. Selenium also helps dislodge mercury, aiding in its elimination. NukeProtect is an ideal selenium-based supplement for purging mercury. Take two capsules daily. Also, take a natural-source vitamin C, such as Purely-C, two capsules twice daily. Take Garlex, 10 drops twice daily.

11 to 18 Points Mild but significant mercury intoxication:
Any excess of mercury in the body is damaging. Attempt to remove this noxious substance through safe means. Mercury is a cellular poison, which binds to human proteins, such as enzymes and cell walls. It easily dissolves in fatty tissues, especially the brain, spinal cord, and nerve sheaths. There, it greatly interferes with nerve cell function, leading to a wide range of neurological diseases and symptoms. The mercury

must be cleansed from the body through a safe means. Nutritional deficiency weakens the body, making it more vulnerable to accumulating mercury. Selenium deficiency is associated with a high risk of mercury contamination. This mineral helps dislodge mercury from cells. As a source of naturally bound selenium take NukeProtect, 2 to 4 capsules twice daily. Also, take the Garlex, 20 drops twice daily. Wild greens assist in mercury removal. Take the GreensFlush made from raw wild edible greens, 10 to 20 drops twice daily. Zinc aids in the reversal of mercury-related cell damage: take 75 mg daily. Vitamin C helps purge mercury. Take also crude natural-source vitamin C, such as Purely-C, 4 to 6 capsules daily. Crude currant extract is a tremendous tonic for detoxification, especially of heavy metals. Currant-C is organic and crude: it is super-rich in natural vitamin C, organic acids, and flavonoids: drink 4 ounces daily. The GreensFlush helps purge mercury: take 20 to 40 drops twice daily. Resvital is rich in natural tartaric acid: take one or two teaspoons daily. Also, mercury and other heavy metals must be cleansed from the water. This can be achieved with a high quality water treatment unit. The finest is made by LifeSource Water Systems. To talk to a sales representative call 1-800-992-3997. Regarding amalgam fillings, consider having them removed. See a competent dentist experienced in their removal.

A heavy metal foot patch would prove invaluable. Only the Kinotakara patch has been proven both safe and effective. In the United States this may only be purchased by mail order: 1-800-243-5242. In Canada it may be purchased from distributors: call 1-866-drspice. This patch directly pulls mercury out of the body as well as other heavy metals/toxins. The mercury is visible as small red spots. Use only Kinotakara. Do not accept imitations. Follow instructions until toxins are cleansed.

19 to 28 Points Moderate and significant mercury intoxication: Any excess of mercury in the body is damaging. Attempt to remove this noxious substance through safe means. Mercury is a cellular poison, which binds to human proteins, such as enzymes and cell walls. It easily dissolves in fatty tissues, especially the brain, spinal cord, and nerve sheaths. There, it greatly interferes with nerve cell function, leading to a wide range of neurological diseases and symptoms. The mercury must be cleansed from the body through a safe means. Nutritional deficiency weakens the body, making it more vulnerable to accumulating mercury. Selenium deficiency is associated with a high risk of mercury contamination. This mineral helps dislodge mercury from cells. The ideal form of this mineral is as a kelp and iodine complex. This is available through the NukeProtect capsules: this supplies selenium plus crude kelp and iodine—take three capsules three times daily. Fat soluble thiamine is needed: take 300 mg daily. Or, for a truly natural source of fat soluble thiamine take Nutri-Sense powder, three heaping tablespoons once or twice daily. Zinc helps the cells of the nervous system heal as a result of mercury poisoning: take 75 mg daily.

Vitamin C helps purge mercury. Take a crude natural-source vitamin C, such as Purely-C, 6 capsules daily. Crude currant extract is a tremendous tonic for detoxification, especially of heavy metals. Currant-C is organic and crude: it is super-rich in natural vitamin C, organic acids, and flavonoids: drink 4 ounces daily. Resvital is a rich source of the metal-chelating substance tartaric acid: take 2 to 3 teaspoons daily. The GreensFlush purges mercury from the bloodstream and liver; take 20 to 40 drops twice daily. LivaClenz, which is rich in oil of cilantro, that is coriander oil, is an effective mercury chelator: take 20 to 40 drops twice daily. Also, take Garlex, 40 drops twice daily.

Mercury and other heavy metal residues should be cleansed from tap water. These metals can even be absorbed through the skin. The finest water purification system is made by LifeSource Water Systems. To talk to a sales representative call 1-800-992-3997.

A heavy metal foot patch would prove invaluable. Only the Kinotakara patch has been proven by research to be both safe and effective. In the United States this may only be purchased by mail order: 1-800-243-5242. In Canada it may be purchased from distributors: call 1-866-drspice. This patch directly pulls mercury out of the body as well as other heavy metals/toxins. The mercury is visible as small red spots. Use only Kinotakara. Do not accept imitations. Follow instructions until toxins are cleansed.

29 to 39 Severe mercury intoxication:
This degree of mercury intoxication is likely inducing significant damage in the tissues. Attempt to remove this noxious substance through a safe means. Mercury is a cellular poison, which binds to human proteins, such as enzymes and cell walls. It blocks enzymes from functioning. It easily dissolves in fatty tissues, especially the brain, spinal cord, and nerve sheaths. There, it greatly interferes with nerve cell function, leading to a wide range of neurological diseases and symptoms. Selenium is the major nutrient which antagonizes mercury. It helps dislodge it from its cellular attachments. The ideal form of this mineral is as a kelp and iodine complex. This is available through the NukeProtect capsules: this supplies selenium plus crude kelp and iodine—take four capsules three times daily. Fat soluble thiamine is needed: take 400 mg daily. Or, for a truly natural source of fat soluble thiamine take Nutri-Sense powder, three heaping tablespoons once or twice daily. Zinc aids in the healing of mercury-damaged cells: take 75 mg daily.

Vitamin C helps purge mercury. Take a crude natural-source vitamin C, such as Purely-C, 4 capsules two or three times daily. Take also crude black currant juice as a source of acidic flavonoids and natural vitamin C: drink unsweetened organic currant juice (that is Currant-C), 4 ounces twice daily. Drink also fresh organic grapefruit juice, 8 ounces twice daily. Red sour grape powder is one of the most aggressive of all sour agents. It is rich in tartaric and malic acid, which are heavy metal binders. Take a heaping teaspoon twice daily in juice or water (ideally, add this to grapefruit or orange juice). As a source of natural cleansing enzymes take ZymaClenz, 2 or 3 capsules twice daily on an empty stomach.

There is a need to cleanse the tap water of mercury and other heavy metals. These metals may be even absorbed through the skin. LifeSource offers the highest quality in home water cleansing systems, featuring high grade activated carbon. This uses state-of-the-art technology to remove heavy metals. To speak to a sales representative call 1-800-992-3997. Use water that is purified or drink high quality mineral water. Do not drink unfiltered tap water. Avoid the intake of refined sugar. The sugar leaches mercury from the fillings, increasing the degree of poisoning.

The GreensFlush helps purge heavy metals. Take three droppersful under the tongue twice daily. This helps extract the heavy metals from the liver as well as blood. Also, take Garlex, 40 or more drops twice daily. What's more, take the Cilantro-plus, 20 or more drops twice daily.

A heavy metal foot patch would prove invaluable. Only the Kinotakara patch has been proven both safe and effective. In the United States this may only be purchased mail order: 1-800-243-5242. In Canada it may be purchased from distributors: call 1-866-drspice. This patch directly pulls mercury out of the body as well as other heavy metals/toxins. The mercury is visible as small red spots. Use only Kinotakara. Do not accept imitations. Follow instructions until toxins are cleansed.

40 to 49 Extreme mercury intoxication:

Warning, this degree of intoxication is causing severe tissue damage. This is why you have such a wide number of symptoms. Mercury is highly toxic to the tissues. It aggressively binds to protein, plus it is easily absorbed into fatty tissues, like the brain and spinal cord. The heart is also fatty, so it easily enters this organ. It causes oxidative damage of the heart and arteries and is a major cause of heart attacks and strokes. Mercury also damages the immune system: a reduced white count may indicate mercury poisoning. This metal poisons the immune cells, greatly reducing their ability to do their work. The mercury binds to the white cells, causing them to lose their normal fluid and amoeba-like actions. As a result, the white cell membranes become brittle or stiff, and they break down easily. Mercury is also deposited in the kidneys and to a lesser degree in the liver. Cleansing these organs of the mineral results in improved health. Selenium is a key substance for cleansing. Organic and/or amino acid chelate selenium is the safe type to use. As a source of organic selenium plus iodine take NukeProtect, four or more capsules three times daily.

Natural vitamin C helps purge mercury from the body through the kidneys and stools. The crude natural vitamin C is the most potent form available, that is for mobilizing toxic metals. Take the Purely-C, four or more capsules four times daily. The crude C has flavonoids, which also block mercury toxicity. Crude currant juice is rich in organic acids and natural vitamin C, which are ideal for cleansing. The organic type is known as Currant-C: drink a bottle daily. Currant-C is a potent intestinal and kidney cleansing tonic and is completely safe for all ages. Take also an agent for purging the liver. The best is the

GreensFlush made from raw wild dandelion and nettle. This is a potent liver detoxification agent: take 40 drops two or more times daily. Mix the GreensFlush in a double shot glass of extra virgin olive oil. Use large amounts of vinegar; it's potent also, because it has the chelating agent acetic acid. Add it to all salads and foods; add two tablespoons to the GreensFlush/olive oil mixture. The acetic acid helps flush the mercury out of the body. Oil of cumin is an excellent agent for cleansing the liver of heavy metals: take 20 drops twice daily (may be added to the flush mixture). Also, take Cilantro-plus: this is extensively used by physicians for mercury detoxification. Take 40 drops of the Cilantro-plus (oil of wild cilantro) twice daily (may also be added to the olive oil flush). Onions and garlic are mercury cleansers. They contain sulfur groups, which bind to this metal. Eat as much of these foods daily as possible, either raw or cooked. Make a garlic/onion/chicken broth and add a few drops of the oil of cumin and cilantro; drink two or three cups daily. As a source of natural cleansing enzymes take Inflam-eez, 4 capsules three times daily on an empty stomach. Also, take Garlex, 40 or more drops twice daily.

If you have dental mercury/silver fillings, they may need to be evaluated as a source of leaching mercury. See a competent naturally inclined dentist for evaluation. Special procedures exist for the removal of these fillings, as they are regarded as hazardous wastes. Avoid the intake of refined sugar. The sugar leaches mercury from the fillings, increasing the degree of poisoning. Plus, it encourages the overgrowth of yeasts, which flourish in the dental tissues.

The GreensFlush helps purge heavy metals. Take three to four droppersful under the tongue twice daily. This helps extract the heavy metals from the liver as well as blood.

A heavy metal foot patch would prove invaluable. Only the Kinotakara patch has been proven by research to be both safe and effective. In the United States this may only be purchased mail order: 1-800-243-5242. In Canada it may be purchased from distributors: call 1-866-drspice. This patch directly pulls mercury out of the body as well as other heavy metals/toxins. The mercury is visible as small red spots. Use only Kinotakara. Do not accept imitations. Follow instructions until toxins are cleansed.

50 and above Profoundly extreme mercury intoxication:

Warning, this degree of intoxication is causing severe tissue damage. This is why you have such a wide number of symptoms. This metal aggressively dissolves in fatty tissues, especially the fatty nervous system, which is the brain, spinal cord, and nerve sheaths. There, it binds to cell proteins, causing damage and death. It also readily poisons the heart and arteries; the heart has a large amount of fat, so mercury dissolves into it. It causes oxidative damage of the heart and arteries and is a major cause of heart attacks and strokes. Mercury also damages the immune system: a reduced white count may indicate mercury poisoning. This metal poisons the immune cells, greatly reducing their ability to do their work. The mercury binds to the white cells, causing them to lose their normal fluid and amoeba-like actions. As a result, the white cell membranes become brittle or stiff, and they break down easily.

Mercury is also deposited in the kidneys and to a lesser degree in the liver. Purging these organs of this toxic metal improves overall health. Selenium is a key substance for this cleansing. Organic and/or amino acid chelate selenium is the safe type to use. This is found in the nutritional supplement NukeProtect. This is an organic yeast and iodine formula, ideal for antagonizing the mercury. Take four capsules of NukeProtect three times daily. This amount is safe to take for three to four months, then reduce the amount to three capsules twice daily. Take also vitamin C, which aids in mercury detoxification. The crude natural vitamin C is most effective. Take Purely-C, 4 or more capsules four times daily. Crude currant juice is rich in organic acids and natural vitamin C, which are ideal for cleansing. The organic type is known as Currant-C: drink a bottle daily. Currant-C is a potent intestinal and kidney cleansing tonic and is completely safe for all ages. Take also an agent for purging the liver. The best is the GreensFlush, which is made from raw wild dandelion and nettles. This is a potent liver detoxification agent: take 40 or more drops three times daily. Mix the GreensFlush with a double shot glass of extra virgin olive oil.

Use large amounts of vinegar; it's potent also, because it has the chelating agent, acetic acid. Add it to all salads and foods; add two tablespoons to the GreensFlush/olive oil mixture. The acetic acid helps flush the mercury out of the body.

Oil of Cilantro-plus is a special type of oil of cilantro. This is extensively used by physicians for mercury detoxification. Take 40 to 80 drops of the oil of Cilantro-plus twice daily. This may also be added to the olive oil flush. Onions and garlic are mercury cleansers. They contain sulfur groups, which bind this metal. Eat as much of these foods daily as possible, either raw or cooked. Make a garlic/onion/chicken broth and add a few drops of the oil of cumin and cilantro; drink two or three cups daily. It halts oxidative damage of the heart and arteries and is a major cause of heart attacks and strokes. Also, take Garlex, 40 drops twice daily.

Mercury also damages the immune system: a reduced white count may indicate mercury poisoning. This metal poisons the immune cells, greatly reducing their ability to do their work. The mercury binds to the white cells, causing them to lose their normal fluid and ameba-like actions. As a result, the white cell membranes become brittle or stiff, and, thus, they easily break down. Mercury is also deposited in the kidneys and to a lesser degree the liver. Cleansing these organs of the mineral results in improved health. Selenium is a key substance for cleansing. Organic and/or amino acid chelate selenium is the safe type to use.

Crude red grape powder is also a critical toxic metal cleanser. It is rich in the natural organic acids, like tartaric and malic acid, which help bind and cleanse metals. This is known as Resvital. Take two or more teaspoons twice daily as an aggressive and natural cleansing agent.

Regarding amalgam fillings, they must be removed. See a competent dentist experienced in their removal. At this degree of mercury overload, the fillings must be carefully removed. Also, avoid the intake of refined sugar. The sugar solubulizes the mercury from dental fillings, increasing the degree of mercury poisoning. Plus, sugar destroys the immune system. It also causes the overgrowth of yeasts, which infest the dental tissues as well as the internal organs. Refined sugar also feeds fungal infestation. Note: it is the highly refined type of sugar that is dangerous.

A heavy metal foot patch would prove invaluable. Only the Kinotakara patch has been proven by research to be both safe and effective. In the United States this may only be purchased mail order: 1-800-243-5242. In Canada it may be purchased from distributors: call 1-866-drspice. This patch directly pulls mercury out of the body as well as other heavy metals/toxins. The mercury is visible as small red spots. Use only Kinotakara. Do not accept imitations. Follow instructions until toxins are cleansed.

Chapter 7
Cancer: A Viral Disease?

Viruses are dangerous entities. They wreak havoc on cellular functions, disrupting metabolism, damaging cell structures, and altering cellular genetics. Over time they cause a vast degree of cell damage and inflammation, readily causing cell death. This damage may lead to a variety of diseases, including cancer.

Certain viruses are known as cancer causing, or in medical terminology, tumorigenic. These viruses infiltrate the inner mechanisms of cells. Here, they use their specialized capacities for invasion to create disease. Viruses have immense powers to infiltrate cells. Once they do so they directly attack the cells' nuclei, where they capitalize on the genetic material. Once established, they use the cells' genetics to replicate themselves. In essence, viruses steal the cells' genes, making these genes work for them instead. This is the kind of 'gene warfare' which develops within virally infected cells. As with any kind of warfare mass chaos, that is destruction, occurs. If the genetic warfare continues unchecked, the natural cell cycle is fully disrupted. The germ takes control of the cell and poisons it. This may lead to mutations and, ultimately, cancer.

Experts agree that at a minimum some 30% of all cancers are infective. It is reasonable to estimate that over one-half of all cancers have a primary infectious cause. Even this estimate may be conservative. Examples of cancers with a definite infectious cause include stomach and duodenal cancers, leukemia, Kaposi's sarcoma, cervical cancer, lymphoma, cancer of the liver, melanoma, mycoses fungoides, prostate cancer, lung cancer, bladder, ovarian, and colon cancer. What's more, inflammatory breast cancer is always infective. Even skin cancer may have an infectious root.

Cervical cancer is an obvious proof of the infectious connection. In this disease virtually all cases are due to a specific infection: the cervical wart (papilloma) virus. It was G. Tortolero-Luna, M.D., who stated that, incredibly, in all cases "in order to have the cancer, you have to have the virus." Liver cancer is also due largely to infection. This is primarily due to the various hepatitis viruses, particularly hepatitis B and C. The viruses directly integrate themselves into the liver cells, in other words, the viral genetic material becomes spliced into the genes of the liver cells, ultimately converting them into cancer cells. Essentially, the virus causes the cells to grow wildly, and a tumor forms. This ultimately destroys the liver as well as the rest of the body.

Viruses cause mutations. This is how they take over the body and, ultimately, destroy it. The cure is simple. The virus must be killed.

Lymphoma is also caused by viral infection, although a variety of other factors, including fungal infestations, toxic chemical exposure, and wrong diet, play a role. Numerous viruses have been found within lymphoma tissue, including SV40, Epstein-Barr virus, and human herpesvirus-8 (HHV-8). Such viruses induce the very mutations in such tissue that lead to cancer. Thus, regarding lymphoma viruses are causative. Again, to cure the lymphoma the viruses must be killed. This is achieved through the intake of potent spice extracts, particularly the multiple spice OregaBiotic capsules, the P73 oil of wild oregano. This combination can readily eradicate the vaccine viruses, effectively purging them from the tissues.

The evidence for SV40 virus infection in humans is compelling, in fact, definite. As reported in *The Lancet* a team of scientists at Baylor College of Medicine provided firm documentation of the infection. The researchers analyzed samples from some 150 patients who had lymphomas and found that over 40% were positive for this germ. In contrast, the majority of the control samples were negative. Say the investigators, "This study further demonstrates that humans can be infected by SV40, an infection that was not suspected in the past..." Concerned about the high incidence of the virus in lymphatic tissue, the researchers speculated on the cause of the spread among humans, claiming that such a spread is occurring in ways which are unclear. Other cancers which contain this virus include tumors of the lining of the intestines, brain tumors (benign and malignant), bone cancers, and mesotheliomas.

It was Dr. Adi Gazdar of Dallas's University of Texas Southwestern Medical School, who confirmed the presence of SV40 in this disease. His study also appears in the March 9 issue of *The Lancet*. Thus, there are a plethora of studies which confirm the unfathomable: that tens of millions of Westerners, in fact, potentially billions of people globally, have been infected with cancer-causing viruses—all as a result of greedy corporate and government policies. This will lead to uncountable deaths from a wide range of diseases, including neurological disorders—multiple sclerosis, Guillain Barré syndrome, Alzheimer's disease, Parkinson's disease, and ALS as well as, of course, cancer. The fact is multiple sclerosis and Guillain Barré syndrome may be a form of polio:

It may also be pointed out that, however dead the virus may be, the giving of any kind of inoculation is likely to precipitate...polio...in a relatively small number of children who perhaps are already harboring the virus. One is led to believe that these dangers are less than the benefits of protection, but when the prediction is by no means 100%, the merits of the method and its statistics become debatable... When...polio...is precipitated by an inoculation the natural defenses of the nervous system seem to be ineffective, and nearly all such illnesses develop into a paralytic form of the disease affecting especially the limb used for the injection.

Contamination, cancer viruses, and more

Today, vaccine manufacture has made no advances. The same dangerous methods are being used when the industry originated. Bayly's monograph further reveals:

According to a (private) bulletin issued by Lederle (September 1954) they have succeeded in growing a deadly...virus in chick embryos (this is the tiny cell culture which ultimately forms into a chicken: note the work of Virginia Livingston-Wheeler demonstrating a plethora of cancer-causing viruses in these embryos). This particular research is being pursued by Dr. Herald R. Cox, who was Principal Bacteriologist of the United States Public Health Service (now the United States Department of Public Health), and was the originator of the chick-embryo-produced vaccine for Rocky Mountain spotted fever and epidemic typhus fever. This latter vaccine was manufactured in hundreds of millions of doses during the last war for the immunization of all American and Canadian as well as Allied troops and the civilian population in typhus-infected areas. Dr. Cox, now Director of the Virus and

Rickettsial Research Department of Lederle Laboratories, states that, in his opinion, chick embryo "is the ideal tissue for mass producing virus vaccines. The chick embryo is always readily available, cheap, and free from potentially dangerous micro-organisms."

The method is now well standardized. A technician uses a dentist's drill to break a tiny hole through the eggshell. Through this opening another technician injects a small amount of living modified virus with a hypodermic needle. The hole is sealed with collodion and the eggs are placed in an incubator for a certain number of days. Before hatching, the eggs are racked and the living embryos, which are now swarming with tremendous quantities of virus, are removed and "processed" by methods necessary to produce either killed or living modified virus vaccines. Lederle, we are told, has used as many as 14 million eggs a year in the production of various vaccines.

The conflict of interest is obvious: first this researcher works for the U.S. government, then for a pharmaceutical house. He creates a medicine that is sponsored and endorsed by the government, the latter, of course, receiving much of its funding from the drug houses. Therefore, he uses the government to serve his own agenda. Public interest has nothing to do with it. Thus, the production of the chicken embryo-based vaccine cannot be trusted. Rather than a public health issue, the creation of the aforementioned vaccine was a business project. This shows how truly tainted the vaccine industry is to utilize the authority of government to promote a business. This is corruption of the highest degree.

What's more, the methods for vaccine manufacture are themselves grotesque. These rely upon growing and then sacrificing untold millions of chicken embryos. These embryos are minced into a bloody soup. This is a septic soup, made of the blood and guts, as well as feces and urine, of immature chickens from artificially infected embryos. Each embryo is "teeming with viruses" before it is ground up for harvest. Yet, what is rarely mentioned is that it is also teeming with fungi, parasites, and bacteria, while also contaminated with a host of noxious chemicals.

This type of a chicken embryo solution is the source of the majority of modern vaccines, although, still, some vaccines are grown on monkey kidney and testicular tissue. Incredibly, still others are grown on human fetal tissues. In all cases the growth materials become contaminated, fully septic—fully microbially infested. This places human beings at a vast risk for physical and immunological devastation.

Chicken blood is notoriously infected with germs, and this is particularly true of the blood of commercially raised chickens. Here, chickens are fed commercial chow, which is derived from a variety of waste products, including the rendered wastes of dead and diseased animals. Livingston, in her landmark work published in the 1950s through 1980s, demonstrated a variety of hostile germs which are routinely found in chickens. The majority of these germs are cancer-causing. Such germs are also found in commercial vaccines, which, again, are derived from these animals. Again, remember the words of the former Chief Virologist of the FDA, J. Anthony Morris, that is that the flu vaccine is carcinogenic. This is largely due to the cancer-causing poultry viruses it contains. It can also be due to the additives formaldehyde and thimerasol, which are carcinogenic.

Commercial chickens surely are a poor source for a public medicine. Such chickens are routinely fed chow which is derived from animal carcasses. The dead animals represent hundreds of species and may include pets, research animals, farm animals, and zoo animals. The wide range of species includes cows, chickens, ducks, pigs, reptiles, rodents, cats, dogs, and deer. The wastes from slaughterhouses are a major component. This includes the blood from slaughtered pigs, cows, calves, chickens, turkeys, and ducks. What's more, dead animals from universities—research animals fed and injected with materials unknown—are also added to the slurry. All such waste is rendered, and the resulting protein and fat is then added to commercial feed. This is then fed to farm animals, mainly pigs and chickens. The blood of the chickens becomes contaminated with a wide range of germs from a vast range of species, and many of these germs are readily transferred into the eggs.

Chapter 8
Guinea Pigs, Dirty Monkeys

Human experimenting is far from new. Through modern medicine since the early 1800s experimentation upon humans has been commonplace. The fact is over this period untold thousands have died as a result of ill-conceived medical experiments. Recall the use in shoe stores of X-rays, as well as the irradiation of the developing thymus glands in children. These experiments with an unknown medical agent, X-rays, lead to thousands of deaths from cancer.

The government and medical profession continuously use people as experimental subjects. Polio experiments were among the first. As early as the 1930s medical researchers dabbled in the concept of a polio vaccine. A number of children had been experimentally inoculated with the vaccine, also produced from monkey tissue. The result was disastrous. Of the 12 children inoculated some five died, while three were severely paralyzed. It was the United State's key public health official, Dr. J. P. Leake, who reported the findings. Writing in the *Journal of the American Medical Association* (1935, 105:2) he notes that after reviewing the findings many physicians will "feel that these cases make undesirable the further use of poliomyelitis virus for human vaccination..." Incredibly, the chemicals used to inactivate the virus are among the most toxic compounds known, sodium ricinoleate, a sodium soap of the castor bean derivative, ricin, and formaldehyde. For obvious reasons both vaccines were abandoned.

Bayly also quotes the authoritative *Medical World News Letter* regarding the nature of the vaccination program. The editors wrote:

> *There is a useful lesson to be learned from the sorry story of the Salk polio vaccine in the U.S.A. It is that a new therapeutic measure of fundamental importance should not be launched until every possible medical and social implication has been considered...Three months ago newspapers throughout he U.S.A. were celebrating one of the greatest medical discoveries of our time and hailing the final conquest of poliomyelitis. Indeed the claims seemed reasonably well substantiated, although more cautious voices were heard over here (that is in Britain). The United States Public Health Service authorized commercial reproduction and relaxed standards of safety testing. In the meantime the tremendous publicity had created a universal demand of the vaccine. Large-scale inoculations were undertaken with results that were catastrophic for a far from negligible number of families. Over 100 cases of poliomyelitis occurred among the vaccinated and, what was more significant, 60 cases among their immediate contacts. There is no doubt that the disease has been propagated by the vaccine. American experts agree that the total elimination of live virus from the cultures may be difficult to secure. These misfortunes would be almost endurable if a whole new generation were to be rendered permanently immune to these. In fact, there is no evidence that any lasting immunity is achieved.*

The question is in light of the aforementioned how could such a vaccine be approved? The researchers have made it clear that rather than preventing polio it caused it. The approval, in fact, was left only to one person: a Dr. Thomas Francis of the University of Michigan. Incredibly, he alone was given the final decision power. Regarding the implementation of a program as critical as a mass vaccination plan, even the inoculation of young children, it is incomprehensible that such a decision would be left to one individual. This is particularly true of an individual who has a vested interest in promoting the program. Francis was Salk's colleague, in fact, teacher. He was intimately involved in the promotion of the polio vaccine plan. Far from independent, emotionally and professionally, he was committed to it. In other words, his life's desire was to ensure the success of such a program. It seems implausible that he would find fault with it. In fact, he would do all in his power to see it through, to find a reason for the correctness of the data, perhaps even to skew it, that is in favor of the approval. Thus, the review process was tainted, there could be no unbiased assessment. Incredibly, millions of individuals were injected and/or orally vaccinated on the basis of faulty research, fully supported by the press and government. This was the greatest experiment upon human beings in the entire world history. What's more, the ultimate consequences have been dire.

No independent party sought to confirm Dr. Francis's findings. It was accepted wholesale, and, incredibly, the plan was immediately placed into action. Within a week of his proclamation of the successful and 'safe' nature of the vaccination—his claim that it was a certain cure for humankind—millions of doses of the vaccine were shipped to centers throughout the country. The fact is well before the official 'approval' the vaccine had been massively produced by a variety of pharmaceutical houses. All of it was strategically prepared well before Dr. Francis's public announcement. He had no choice but to find in favor of it. What's more, surely, if there were unfavorable findings, he would be forced to dismiss them. Thus, he would use his position as intellectual authority to ensure the result.

It would appear that the American public had been duped. Essentially, an entire nation of people had been set up by a government and industry which lacked all independent proof of the safety or efficacy of their plan—no evidence existed that the vaccine would truly help the population or that it could be safely administered. Yet, with great fanfare the vast majority of North Americans were vaccinated. The result was and continues to be a catastrophe beyond comprehension and the development of a vast number of chronic diseases resulted, including a variety of potentially fatal cancers.

Francis and Salk were friends, in fact, colleagues. They co-published papers. They had parties and dinners together. They both worked at the same facilities. Clearly, the Francis review, which led to the launch of the vaccine, was biased. This is never done so openly today, rather, it is disguised. Thus, from the onset the vaccine approval process was fraudulent. Incredibly, the government gave the approval process to the professor of the student—the very man who trained the student to pursue this research. Thus, it was, in essence, Francis's own research which he was approving, the greatest possible conflict of interest conceivable. True, like all professionals there were professional jealousies. Yet, both men had the same goals: to institute national vaccination programs. This was to industrialize invasive medicine. More critically, both had received funding from the same institution, which was pro-vaccine. If despite professional jealousies Francis found against the polio vaccine and Salk's work, surely, his own funding would be at risk. Thus, even if he discovered that the Salk research was faulty, he would be unable to render an unbiased view.

With the backing of Francis, Salk sought to industrialize the vaccine. The objective was to create a national approach that would bring in further grants. Of course, this was paid by the taxpayers. Yet, they concluded that if they could succeed in eradicating such a visible and feared disease, then, they would become famous and rich which would lead to further research contracts. In other words, they could be guaranteed permanent access to public funds. Aaron Klein demonstrates the connection in his book *Trial By Fury: The Polio Vaccine Controversy*, who writes:

> The two virologists published many papers together and sometimes Salk even had his name listed first. The question of whose name is listed first on a publication may seem a trifling matter, but it is as important to a scientist as top billing on a theater marquee to an actor. The implication is that the first-named author has made the most important and greatest contribution to the work even if that is not necessarily the case. After a while professional jealousies began to taint the relationship between the two men. Salk's slow rate of advancement...made him restless, and he began to look around for a situation where he would be free to do whatever research interested him...

Regarding the rush to create a national vaccination plan there was great pressure, not only within researchers' minds for their own purposes but within the government itself. There was a need to create an image of "heroes of humankind" in order to induce public support. There was also a sense of panic arising from the funding organizations. Regarding the status of polio in the post-war era says Klein:

> At the end of World War II the men on the board of the National Foundation for Infantile Paralysis (were) found restless, confused, and without direction...major attention was on the events of the war and not on the publicity tactics of Basil O'Connor. With the death of Franklin Roosevelt...the foundation lost its big symbol but still had his memory to exploit. Research specifically relevant to the polio problem had lagged during the war, and the foundation people were not quite sure just how to start things up again to their best advantage.

> The foundation had been generous with grants, and several institutions, such as the Johns Hopkins School of Public Health, had received long-term grants...well into the millions of dollars. (For instance, the) work of Francis on influenza was one example (the very man who was given the vaccine data to approve). Among...virologists, the foundation came to be known as a ready source of grant money, which benefited the scientists as well as the scientific establishments (that is the universities)...Meanwhile the number of polio cases was increasing, and money was needed to take care of the victims in addition to money needed for research. The "significant breakthroughs" upon which the foundation fundraisers relied to inspire the public to greater giving were non-existent. The foundation still depended on the (public) for its sustenance, and the public was fickle. A fair amount of money was still collected, but much of it was from habitual givers, those people who automatically deposited their change in the little boxes that bore the pathetic pictures of paralyzed children in braces and wheelchairs. Giving money to conquer

polio was the thing to do. It was part of the mother-and-the-flag national mystique, and not to give was considered somewhat "unpatriotic."

Thus, it is easy to see the unscientific nature, in fact, emotionally charged basis, of this approach. The unprecedented rush to the vaccine is further confirmed by the following:

O'Conner was well aware that even this trickle of dimes and quarters could dry up—if something exciting did not happen soon. He had always relied on press releases that contained such phrases as "encouraging development" to keep the public in a giving mood even though he ran the risk of receiving angry letters from embarrassed scientists. O'Connor assumed even more risk of angering scientists when, in 1946, a semi-retired virologist, Harry Weaver, was appointed Director of Research in an attempt to launch a concerted research effort. The risk to O'Connor lay in what was implied in Weaver's title. Scientists have never liked to be directed, but O'Connor felt that he had waited long enough for scientists to eliminate polio with their individual uncoordinated efforts. Direction was needed, engineered in such a way that the independent-minded scientists would not know they were being directed. That was Harry Weaver's job.

The Johns Hopkins School of Public Heath and Hygiene had long been one of the biggest beneficiaries of the foundation, receiving millions of dollars in donations. This was from generous gifting from the public. There, Bodian, Howe, and Morgan attempted to immunize monkeys with inactivated polio virus preparations. Some of these monkeys survived challenges with live polio virus and others did not. This work not only pointed to possibilities of killed-virus polio vaccines but also indicated that there was probably more than one type of polio virus. Further work suggested that there were three main types of polio virus, but neither the Johns Hopkins group nor anyone else could be absolutely sure of this. There could be four, five, ten, twenty, or an unlimited number of such viruses, plus in any monkey or serum there could be other species unknown. The failures indicated that there must be in any preparation dozens of viruses. Thus, it was clear that any proposed polio vaccine would have to be effective against all types of polio virus.

Ultimately, the vaccine became a massive business project. Salk was a mere laborer. As further documentation that Salk was a mere figurehead for a broader agenda Klein notes:

> Before a truly effective polio vaccine could be considered...all the known strains of polio viruses had to be typed...Typing viruses was not particularly exciting work. It was the kind of job usually given to a graduate assistant or to a technician. A virologist who thought much of himself was not likely to volunteer to spend several years running typing tests on literally thousands of known polio strains, not to mention the new ones that keep cropping up. Typing viruses was dull, tedious work and not the stuff of which Nobel Prizes were made...One of the men who came to Weaver's attention was Jonas Salk, who was working on flu virus at Pittsburgh. Salk had no experience with polio virus, but that was good, since he was less likely to be encumbered with orthodox notions.
>
> Salk eagerly accepted Weaver's suggestion...The foundation...organized a Typing Committee to oversee the work of Salk...The committee was made up of many of the major figures in virology, such as

Albert Sabin, Thomas Francis, David Bodian, John Paul, and William Hammon, the men who would not give any of their own time to the actual typing. As members of the committee they understood that their job was to tell the virus typers how to do their work. It was further understood that Salk and the others would do exactly as they were told.

As the project wore on, Salk found that he had less and less time to spend in the laboratory, for more and more time was required at his desk. He had to attend to problems of budget, ordering supplies and renewing grants. At times he was little more than a monkey-keeper. Monkeys were the mainstay of polio research. At the time they were the only known, readily available animals susceptible to all types of polio, and that was unfortunate for polio researchers. Monkeys were expensive to buy, difficult to maintain, and took up a great deal of room in the laboratory. They were much more difficult to handle than the duller rabbits and mice. Monkeys, nasty-tempered, especially the widely used Rhesus monkey, could inflict vicious bites. In 1935 a promising young bacteriologist, William Brebner, was bitten by a monkey and died of a "paralytic disease".

In captivity the habits of monkeys cannot be described as clean, and housebreaking is an unknown concept in connection with them. They have a rather disconcerting habit of defecating into their hands and throwing the excrement at passers-by. Any qualms at the "inhumanity" of injecting viruses into the spinal cords of these "cute" creatures, who look so much like little people, is soon dispelled by their many annoying attributes.

Yet, incredibly, there would have been no such annoying attributes were it not for the fact that these creatures were held against their will in confinement in utterly "inhumane" surroundings. In the wild these creatures roam the bush—they thrive on a wide range, utter freedom. There they do not toss feces at passers-by, nor do they defecate in their hands.

The monkeys were brought to an environment which was totally foreign. This could only lead to disease. What's more, they were under great stress. In nature they were free, and now they were caged. Klein continued:

> The monkeys had to be imported from Southeast Asia, and many of them died from respiratory ailments...It was frequently necessary to expend time and money in nursing the animals back to health before they could be used. There were so many casualties that the foundation decided to go into the monkey business. A monkey farm was set up in South Carolina, and this operation supplied polio researchers with most of the monkeys they needed.

Yet, there were a variety of other dangerous short cuts, and "monkey business" which were taken to further the agenda, that is the goals of power, glory, and money:

> The actual work of typing viruses went very quickly, primarily because faster methods were adopted...(by) Salk, in spite of the establishment's instructions. Salk was quickly bored with the mechanics of this work, and long before the project was finished, he was looking for other things to do.
>
> Jonas Salk (was) caught up in the excitement (about developing a polio vaccine)...and Sabin made no secret of his desire to be the latter-day Pasteur. Salk, Sabin, the

Johns Hopkins people, and most of the country's virologists looked to the foundation for support...

In other words, rather than humanitarian concerns these men sought fame and fortune. This made them dangerous. Thus, it is no surprise that they created an international epidemic. This epidemic has caused unmerciful pain and torment as well as the loss of uncountable lives. These were far from the saviors of humanity, as they were commonly supposed. They were merely greedy, recognition-oriented scientists, whose purposes were self gain. Thus, they took short cuts, which cost human lives and welfare. This is demonstrated by the fact that for a number of scientists there was a mad race to gain notoriety for the cure—to achieve not necessarily the best or safest medicine but, rather, first place—and, therefore, a vested position for funding:

> *Even before the revelations of Enders and Bodian two virologists, Herald Cox and Hilary Koprowski, had been working on an attenuated vaccine. Their situation was much different from that of Salk and Sabin. They were in the employ of the Lederle Division of the American Cyanamid Company, one of the largest pharmaceutical manufacturers in the world, and their money and support came from the company. Their situation at Lederle was unique. Never before had a commercial enterprise so committed itself to the development of a vaccine from scratch. Usually a pharmaceutical concern would provide its resources for the manufacture of a vaccine or similar medication after the basic research, which had been done elsewhere.*
>
> *Cox and Koprowski were definite contenders for vaccine honors, and the virologists who presented vaccine proposals to the foundation did so in the*

knowledge that the pair at Lederle could very well get there first. The competition was...a race...and the foundation did not want to be second.

Thus, succeeding at quickly bringing a vaccine to market was more critical to the powers-to-be than reproducible science. Safety, while a factor, was neglected—it was a who-will-be-first focus, and if safety must be compromised, so be it.

Salk himself was always in a hurry. It was well known that he was highly impatient. He was obsessed, relentlessly pursuing a conclusion for his work. Under the employ of the foundation it was Salk who brazenly pursued the use of monkeys as a tissue source. It was he, along with Sabin, who popularized the use of monkey testicular and kidney cells as the growth media for the cells despite the fact that the latter are notoriously contaminated with germs.

Salk never seemed to consider the possibility that the vaccines were thoroughly contaminated. Apparently, he gave no thought to the monumentally contaminated organs of the creatures: their kidneys and testes. He failed to sufficiently test the vaccine solutions to rule out contaminants that could prove fatal or cause disease. At one time he had even planned to add the vaccine to a common fluid, incredibly, monkey kidney and testicular serum added to eggnog or milk. This he would conveniently give to children as the preferred medium.

Such an approach is inconceivable—to add a chemical-laden septic fluid to common foods. Yet his plan was superceded by Koprowski, another harried scientist, who 'fed' the vaccine to unwitting children via chocolate milk. The victims were, in fact, mentally retarded children from a New York State institution. Experts at the time condemned this test as dangerous and unethical, yet, Koprowski was never held accountable. Obviously, such men lacked any moral basis for their theories and had little or no interest in public safety.

Salk continued working on his vaccine, settling on the use of formaldehyde as the inactivating agent. Yet, the use of formaldehyde as a sterilizing agent raised great concerns among researchers. This was because of the Brodie catastrophe, where in 1935 children given formaldehyde-treated vaccines died, which meant that the virus had survived. One well respected colleague, John Enders, reportedly referred to Salk's work as quackery. The final results proved Enders prophetic.

Salk's work was based largely on trial and error. This was certainly true of the use of formaldehyde. Here, it was determined that the 'right' dose was 1:250, that is one part of formaldehyde for every 250 parts of virus. This was no guarantee of sterilization: it was merely an educated guess. After exposing the virus to this concentration there now remained the crucial challenge of determining if any viruses survived. One way of doing this was to inject the virus material into monkeys, particularly into their brains. Here, investigators assumed that if the virus was still infective, an obvious illness, frank polio complete with paralysis, would result. Yet, according to Klein regarding animal testing as a proof for safety and effectiveness:

> ...results could never be certain. Monkeys are not people...One could never be certain that a batch of virus harmless to a monkey would not paralyze a human. There was always the possibility of a few live virus particles slipping undetected into a given batch of vaccine.

Yet, despite such concerns Salk proceeded aggressively, producing huge batches of vaccine solutions. He then tested each batch on monkeys to see if polio would develop.

Monkeys injected with killed-virus stayed alive, with high blood antibody levels, and successfully resisted challenge with live, virulent virus. In order to be injected, the virus had to be suspended in a liquid. Salk chose mineral oil, which served as an adjuvant—that is it seemed to enhance the effect of the vaccine. The mineral oil held on to the virus at the injection site for a while before releasing it bit by bit. There was much disagreement over the use of adjuvants. Many thought they were too irritating and could even initiate cancers. Others were concerned that the use of viruses grown in monkey kidney tissue might damage the recipient's kidneys.

However, the March of Dimes' media machinery was now in high gear, revealing to the world the "tremendous progress" made by a "young man in Pittsburgh." Attending was a news columnist who specialized in scandal-driven stories. He launched an article headed, "New Polio Vaccine—Big Hopes Seen." The result was precisely the opposite of what any true scientist would desire. Says Klein:

> Now everything that everybody did not want to happen happened. Parents started to demand the vaccine from their doctors, and virologists and other scientists chided Salk for being a publicity-seeker, which was...devastating...

Yet, if the aforementioned were true why were such media hounds invited to the session? The fact is the vaccine proponents generated this national, rather, international, exposure. As confirmed by a recent article in *The Chicago Tribune* (April 12, 2005) Salk was largely a glory seeker. He always wanted to surround himself in the limelight. With fame comes riches, whether in direct profits or 'scientific' grants. Without such notoriety the advancement of a career is stalled. Surely, in the case of the polio vaccine the seeking of personal gain muddied the acclaimed purpose: to help the suffering masses.

Yet, the publicity surrounding this purported cure was far from Salk's own doing. There were other self-serving forces, notably the March of Dimes, as well as reporters, who sought personal gain, while failing to consider the implications. What if the vaccine eventually proved unsafe? What would the long-term consequences be? Should fame, fortune, and the procurement of funding come before human safety and the safety of innocent children? In the case of the polio vaccine personal desires superceded safety, and, as a result, today, tens of millions of people suffer the consequences. The March of Dimes and its unabashed promoter, O'Conner, wanted to maintain its vicious grip on public donations. Salk desired to win the race for notoriety as well as maintain steady funding. Sabin, whose needs for recognition were legendary, publically desired to become the modern-day Pasteur. Salk, Sabin, and the March of Dimes, as well as the Salk vaccine reviewer, Francis, sought to establish a firm connection to funding. The taxpayer-funded polio vaccine was the medium to achieve this: at any cost, even the cost of human lives.

People may have a hard time believing this, that there would be vicious intent—that people would disregard the needs of human beings in their pursuits. "If the government approves it", people believe, "it must be good." Yet, the question arises, what is the government? Is it a means to serve the people, or the tool for self-centered interests, controlled by autocrats, who seek only their own personal agenda. It must be remembered that it is lawyers who rule the government. Under the typical circumstances people distrust lawyers. Why would it change for lawyer-politicians? The fact is well known that lawyers enact laws for their own benefit, for the purposes of the special interest club, not for the people in general.

So it was for the government and its involvement with the vaccine. It foisted the polio vaccine upon the people for its own purposes. The U.S. government, while promoting this therapy, never tested it to ensure its safety. Also no action was taken after it was deemed unsafe, that is after numerous people died and became paralyzed. Despite its endorsement the government failed to perform even a single independent trial. Rather, it relied upon the manufacturers' data. As mentioned previously the State of Idaho invited the government to inspect the people felled and crippled by the vaccine. The State took action, cancelling any further vaccines. The Federal government failed to take action, refusing to investigate the debacle.

Regarding the Salk vaccine there was plenty of opposition. A number of prominent scientists disputed the claims for safety. They were concerned about the aggressive nature of the types of polio viruses he used, one of which, the Mahoney Strain, was highly destructive. This strain was one of the most pathogenic strains of viruses known, which vigorously attacked the spinal column and brain. Incredibly, it was the primary strain used by Salk. The effectiveness of formaldehyde in killing the virus had already come under question. In fact, previous research had proven it faulty.

Sabin and Enders, though, admittedly, in competition with Salk, deemed the entire project as "a ghastly mistake." They recognized the dangers of the Mahoney strain and were skeptical of Salk's inactivation technique. However, such objections were not to be considered. The publicity machine was in place. Now, the public demanded the vaccine, insisting on the need for clinical trials. Had the public known the potential dangers, perhaps it wouldn't have been so insistent. Yet, this was not to be. The drug companies made the preparations: an essentially poorly tested vaccination, derived from a most toxic source—the genital and excretory tissues of caged animals—was to be injected into American children. It was now unstoppable.

A special committee consisting of involved parties, as well as scientists, was formed to prepare for the trial. For over a year the committee analyzed the possibilities. Bitter arguing was commonplace. Outside scientists assailed the committee, claiming the entire idea of mass vaccination as unsafe. Due to such concerns outside scientists attempted to duplicate Salk's work, the creation of a supposedly dead vaccine using formaldehyde. Dr. Albert Milzer of the Michael Reese Hospital had most disconcerting results. Using Salk's technique, repeatedly, he kept finding a failure of sterilization. In other words, he kept getting live virus. Regarding this Salk failed to act. The pharmaceutical houses also failed to achieve sterilization. Continuously, they found live vaccine in the chemically treated batches. Yet, the pressure was on. Thus, these concerns were ignored. According to Klein:

> ...the vaccine issue had now left the laboratory and was in the daily papers. There was much at stake. The pharmaceutical houses were getting impatient...(Due to savvy marketing the) public wanted a vaccine in time for the 1954 polio season...

Furthermore, he makes clear the reason for the public push for this vaccination:

> The foundation had brought the public pressure upon itself. For almost twenty years it had built up the image of polio as a national disaster. Summers were periods of dread. Every wimper, sniffle, vague muscle ache, and minor temperature increase in children terrorized parents. The fear had keep the money flowing; now the donors wanted results... The fear of polio, so skillfully promoted by the foundation's advertising, could trigger many reactions... (in the public's aggression)...there would be desperate attempts to get what little vaccine was available.

There was nothing to prevent pharmaceutical houses from utilizing the staff and know-how gathered from working with the Salk preparations to produce their own vaccine and test it in their own laboratories.

Thus, due to these concerns the committee approved a so-called field trial. Quickly, a study design was created, and in only a few months the vaccine was produced. The government now became involved. Due to financial and political pressures the program was allowed to proceed without restrictions. Western and, particularly, American, children were used as guinea pigs and were injected with a vaccine of unknown safety. However, certain scientists at the National Institutes of Health insisted that the vaccine was unsafe and that in order to render it free of pathogens mercury must be added. This was in the form of merthiolate, a deadly poison. Salk resisted the idea, claiming it would reduce the vaccine's effectiveness. However, the government won, and mercury was added to the solution.

There were no safety studies performed to ensure that the injection of mercury, as well as formaldehyde, through vaccines was safe. Nor was there any proof that the vaccine was free of microbial contaminants. Rather, evidence existed that it was grossly contaminated. Yet, the promised deadline arrived, and, thus, the 'experimental' vaccine was injected into approximately 7000 children: American citizens.

There was no means of assuring safety for the vaccine. After all, it was made from the tissues of caged monkeys, who, notoriously, develop disease. There is no means to keep such monkeys hygienic. Rather, it is a violation of hygiene—disease in such creatures is an expected consequence. Drug houses observed the challenges, and due to financial, governmental, and public pressure, pushed through the agenda relentlessly. Safety controls were reprehensible. Unless fulminant polio was found warnings were disregarded. For instance, at government labs after being injected with the Salk vaccine, now made by the drug houses, six test monkeys suddenly died. Incredibly, since autopsies revealed no evidence of polio, the results were ignored. Scientists also became aware that many of the batches of vaccine contained live polio viruses. This was leaked to the press but was quickly dispelled by the foundation's propaganda apparatus. Scientists also raised the issue that mice, when injected with the vaccine, became paralyzed. This too was somehow diffused as a "non-specific" finding.

Perhaps the disregard for human life may be explained by the major forces behind the polio vaccines: chemical companies, for instance, Parke-Davis and American Cyanamid. These corporations produced lethal toxins. Such toxins cause untold damage to the ecosystem and, particularly, to living beings. Such chemical companies have no interest in human safety.

Today, in the Western world the intake or exposure to chemicals, that is drugs, is the primary cause of premature death. Could anyone expect altruism to arise from such companies? It is the lust for profits which rules: safety concerns are routinely neglected and in many instances non-existent. These are the companies which have poisoned the earth killing humans and exterminating entire species. No good could arise from them.

Chemical companies, such as American Cyanamid, could not create noxious chemicals, such as lethal pesticides, and, then, be expected to make 'safe' or chemical-free vaccines. Rather, it would be expected that such productions would be abounding in disease-causing chemicals. The fact is the vaccine would be a way for the chemical company to distribute its productions. Nor could such a company be expected to truly care for human lives. Thus, it is no surprise that the oral polio vaccine made by the former American Cyanamid (now known as Wyeth) is responsible for perhaps the greatest outbreak of cancer ever known in the human race.

American Cyanamid skirted the law and took short cuts to bring its vaccine to market. Thus, it put corporate profits ahead of human safety, creating an international epidemic.

Any statistic can be manipulated. If a company or concern is unhesitant to add deadly poisons to the human body, whether by pill, gross pollution, or injection, why would there be an inhibition for distorting the facts? For the majority of Westerners it is the vaccination program which must be credited for curing polio. It is this program which has saved lives. It could never cause disease. Any other conclusion would be regarded as inaccurate, in fact, radical. Those who claim otherwise would be deemed rabble-rousers, perhaps fanatics.

The government and the medical authorities could not be wrong. The "High Priests" of the universities must tell only the truth. There could never be any corrupt agendas—never any neglect of public interest—never any deliberate attempt to do harm. Yet, even if it isn't deliberate surely there is at a minimum a lack of good sense or more likely an unbridled desire to gain fame and riches: at any expense. What else could explain the idiocy of it all: the use of septic monkey tissues from disease-infested organs and known to be infected, as the source for the vaccine. Anyone with the least degree of common sense would realize the potential consequences: the obvious risk for transmission of disease.

The majority of Westerners suffer at least a degree of vaccine poisoning. The extent to which this occurs may be determined by certain symptoms. Surely, people throughout the globe have been poisoned by these medications. The symptoms of vaccine intoxication are predictable. Take the following test to see if you suffer from vaccine intoxication:

Add up the following points. Which of these applies to you?

Signs/symptoms	Points
1. chronically suppressed immune system	(1)
2. reduced body temperature	(2)
3. failure to mount a strong immune response	(1)
4. failure to mount a fever during infections	(2)
5. always feel cold inside	(2)
6. low white blood cell count	(3)
7. low albumin level	(2)
8. low globulin level	(3)
9. low resistance to infections	(2)
10. readily develop lung infections	(1)
11. chronic intestinal disorders	(1)
12. fibromyalgia-like symptoms	(1)
13. chronic fatigue syndrome	(2)
14. muscle aches, which are persistent	(1)
15. low grade fever	(2)
16. night sweats	(1)
17. chronic stiffness of the spine	(2)
18. multiple joint aches	(1)
19. numbness and tingling	(2)
20. lupus-like symptoms	(1)
21. history of scleroderma	(3)
22. rheumatoid arthritis	(1)
23. muscular dystrophy	(1)
24. myasthenia gravis	(2)
25. autism	(3)
26. attention deficit disorder	(2)
27. multiple sclerosis	(3)
28. Parkinson's disease	(1)
29. Alzheimer's disease	(2)
30. history of several cancers	(2)

31. history of bizarre or unusual brain,
    bone, or lung cancer   (4)
32. history of cancer of the brain, bone,
    or lungs (that is if not a smoker)   (1)
33. history of mesothelioma   (5)
34. readily develop tumors or cancerous growths   (3)
35. constant rigidity of the muscles   (2)
36. constant rapid heartbeat   (1)
37. tremors   (2)
38. seizures/convulsions (or epilepsy)   (2)
39. mental retardation   (2)
40. eczema/psoriasis   (3)
41. lymphoma or leukemia   (3)
42. multiple myeloma   (3)
43. sudden onset of diabetes   (2)
44. thyroid cysts or tumors   (2)
45. swollen lymph nodes   (3)
46. loss of muscle strength   (2)
47. shingles   (1)
48. frequent cold sore outbreaks   (1)
49. Bell's palsy or trigeminal neuralgia   (2)
50. juvenile diabetes (Type 1)   (3)

Your score _____

Evaluation of your score

1 to 6 points Mild vaccine intoxication:
You have a certain degree of damage due to vaccinations. This damage may weaken the immune system, increasing the vulnerability to chronic diseases. The risk for cancer is

increased, as is the risk for the development of neurological conditions as well as joint and muscular diseases. In order to eliminate this risk the body must be purged of vaccine-induced germ residues. This can be achieved with spice extracts, for instance, oil of wild oregano and OregaBiotic. Take five drops of the oil twice daily and a capsule of OregaBiotic twice daily. For further information on purging the tissues of such germs see Appendix A.

7 to 13 points Moderate vaccine intoxication:
You have a significant risk of vaccine toxicity. As a result, you have endured damage to your immune system. This damage significantly increases the risks for the development of chronic or degenerative diseases, particularly inflammatory disorders, cancer, diabetes, heart disorders, and joint/muscular diseases. There is also a significantly increased risk for neurological disorders such as Alzheimer's disease, Parkinson's disease, ALS, multiple sclerosis, muscular dystrophy, Creutzfeld-Jakob Disease (CJD), and myasthenia gravis. Herpetic infections, Bell's palsy, and trigeminal neuralgia are also at a high incidence. All such toxicity may be attributed to the highly noxious effects of vaccines. To eliminate this risk the body must be purged of all vaccine-induced germ residues. This may be achieved through the intake of the oil of wild oregano, notably the edible and highly safe P73 Oreganol and the OregaBiotic. Take 20 or more drops of the Oreganol twice daily and 2 or 3 capsules of the OregaBiotic two or more times daily. Take also the Juice of Oregano, an ounce twice daily. At night take a high quality probiotic (natural bacteria) supplement such as Health-Bac, which is superior in its ability to implant.

A liver cleansing program is also invaluable. Take LivaClenz, 3 capsules twice daily with fat-containing meals. Take also the raw wild GreensFlush, three droppersful twice daily. Also, eat a crude unprocessed raw honey, for instance, Wild Oregano or Mediterranean Wild Flower Honey, two tablespoons daily. For more information regarding purging the tissues of these pathogens see Appendix A.

14 to 24 Severe vaccine intoxication:

Warning, you have an extreme risk of vaccine toxicity. As a result, you have endured damage to your immune system. This damage significantly increases the risks for the development of chronic or degenerative diseases, particularly inflammatory disorders, cancer, diabetes, heart disorders, diabetes, and joint/muscular diseases. There is also a significantly increased risk for neurological disorders such as Alzheimer's disease, Parkinson's disease, ALS, multiple sclerosis, muscular dystrophy, CJD, and myasthenia gravis. There is also a high risk for herpetic infections, Bell's palsy, and trigeminal neuralgia. There is also a high risk for the development of autoimmune disorders, particularly disorders of the endocrine glands. The development of connective tissue diseases, including rheumatoid arthritis, scleroderma, and lupus is likely. All such toxicity may be attributed to the highly noxious effects of vaccines. To eliminate this risk the body must be purged of all vaccine-induced germ residues. This may be achieved through the intake of the oil of wild oregano, notably the edible and highly safe P73 Oreganol, and the OregaBiotic. Take 40 or more drops of the Oreganol twice daily (the SuperStrength is preferable) and 3 capsules of the OregaBiotic three or more times daily. Take also the Juice of Oregano, an ounce or two twice daily. Also, replacing the natural bacteria in the bowel is critical. Take a high grade healthy bacteria supplement, such as Health-Bac, a teaspoon at night in warm water before bedtime. A liver purge is invaluable. Take LivaClenz, 3 capsules twice daily with a fat-containing meal. Take also the wild

GreensFlush, 3 droppersful twice daily. Also, eat a crude unprocessed raw honey, for instance, Wild Oregano or Mediterranean Wild Flower Honey, three tablespoons daily. For more information regarding purging the tissues of these pathogens see Appendix A.

25 and above Extreme vaccine intoxication:
Your risks for physical degeneration are vast. In particular, the risks for the development of cancer, particularly lymphatic cancer and leukemia, are monumental. As a result of the vaccine viruses, particularly the simian virus 40, the immune system has endured extreme damage. This damage significantly increases the risks for the development of chronic or degenerative diseases, particularly inflammatory disorders, cancer, diabetes, heart disorders, and joint/muscular diseases. There is also a significantly increased risk for neurological disorders such as Alzheimer's disease, Parkinson's disease, ALS, multiple sclerosis, muscular dystrophy, CJD, and myasthenia gravis. Herpetic infections, Bell's palsy, and trigeminal neuralgia are also at a high incidence. There is also a high risk for the development of autoimmune disorders, particularly disorders of the endocrine gland, including Addison's disease and Hashimoto's disease.

There is also a high risk for the development of connective tissue diseases, including rheumatoid arthritis, scleroderma, and lupus. All such toxicity may be attributed to the highly noxious effects of vaccines. To eliminate this risk the body must be purged of all germ residues. This may be achieved through the intake of the oil of wild oregano, notably the edible and highly safe P73 Oreganol, and the OregaBiotic. Take 60 or more drops of the Oreganol twice daily (the SuperStrength is preferable) and 3 capsules of the OregaBiotic three or more times daily. Take also the Juice of Oregano, two ounces twice daily. Also, take oil of propolis (Prop-a-Heal), 20 drops twice daily. At night take a high quality probiotic (natural bacteria) supplement such as Health-Bac, which is superior in its ability to implant.

A liver cleansing program is also invaluable. Take LivaClenz, 3 capsules three times daily with fat-containing meals. Take also the wild GreensFlush, three droppersful twice daily. Also, eat a crude unprocessed raw honey, for instance, wild oregano or Mediterranean Wild Flower Honey, three tablespoons daily. For more information regarding purging the tissues of these pathogens see Appendix A.

Vaccines are among the most barbaric of all modern medical procedures. This is largely due to the fact that these are drugs made from animal residues, and such residues are notoriously contaminated. Essentially, contaminants—disease-causing agents—are injected or consumed by the body in order to create a response.

Such an approach could never create good health. What's more, vaccines are based upon poor, perhaps incomplete, science. The use of vaccines is based upon a theory. Why place your life at risk for a baseless approach? It is well known that vaccines, in fact, cause disease, including certain degenerative conditions. Those conditions are far more devastating upon the human race than any of the diseases that vaccines supposedly prevent. Cancer, heart attacks, strokes, brain damage, inflammatory disorders, autoimmune diseases, rheumatoid arthritis, diabetes, and liver disease are all consequences of vaccines. Which is more destructive to humankind: these or measles, mumps, polio, and rubella?

A proven connection?

That vaccines are a major cause of cancer is beyond dispute. This is largely because they introduce a variety of pathogens into the body, which are carcinogenic. These are largely animal pathogens, completely foreign to the human body. These germs agitate human cells, causing toxicity and, therefore, inflammation. The inflammation ultimately leads to genetic damage and, therefore, cancer. Plus, the germs may directly incite cancer. This is because the germs necessarily must overtake cellular operations. Many such germs become incorporated directly into the cell, consuming and overriding the cellular genetics. This must lead to disease as well as tumor formation.

Regarding cancer it is difficult to believe that medical procedures are largely responsible. The idea that physicians or, rather, the pharmaceutical cartel, could be the culprits for such a vast degree of disease, death, and disability seems unfathomable. Yet, much evidence points to this fact. What's more, the connection has long been realized. It was in the early 1900s when an observant medical doctor, W. B. Clarke, made an incredible discovery. He documented a direct connection between tumor formation and vaccinations. Said Clarke,

> *Cancer was practically unknown until compulsory vaccination with cowpox vaccine began to be introduced.*

Yet, based upon his medical observations Clarke made an even more dramatic statement:

> *I have had to deal with two hundred cases of cancer, and I never saw a case of cancer in an unvaccinated person.*

The fact that vaccines introduce cancer-causing germs is beyond dispute. The risk for cancer is dependent upon the degree of germ load. The greater the number of vaccinations a person receives the higher is the risk for cancer development. Yet, it was again Dr. James Howenstine who offered a compelling explanation for this debacle. According to Howenstine:

W. B. Clarke's important observation that cancer was not found in people who fail to get vaccinated demands an explanation and one now appears forthcoming. All vaccines given over a short period of time to an immature immune system deplete the thymus gland (the primary gland involved in immune reactions) of irreplaceable immature immune cells. Each of these cells could have multiplied and developed into an army of valuable cells to combat infection and growth of abnormal cells. When these immune cells have been used up, permanent immunity may not appear. The Arthur Research Foundation in Tucson, Arizona, estimates that up to 60% of our immune system may be exhausted by multiple mass vaccines...(while) only 10% of immune cells are permanently lost when a child is permitted to develop natural immunity...

This is a compelling analysis. Could it be that vaccines are the cause of the monumental epidemic of immune system disorders: chronic fatigue, viral syndrome, fibromyalgia, eczema, asthma, chronic bronchitis, autoimmune disorders, thyroid growths, and more? A 50% or more depletion of the thymus gland is catastrophic. It demonstrates the true mechanism of action of the vaccines: severe immune suppression, in fact, destruction. If the immune system is greatly weakened, it is unable to respond to the typical infections.

What a criminal act it is to deplete the immune system to such a degree. If it is depleted, it will be unable to respond to noxious invaders. If it is overcome, it will be unable to cleanse from the body potential carcinogens. There will no longer be the 'normal' response to germs such as high fever, rash, aches, pains, chills, and sweats. The immune system has become fully depleted and is no longer able to properly respond. Thus, there are no longer the typical childhood diseases with the patterns so commonly recognized before mass vaccination: the expected skin and systemic reactions of chicken pox, mumps, and measles, the powerful chills and fever of strep or staph infections. The entire mechanism of the immune system is disrupted. Thus, vaccines are a kind of drug, which interferes with cellular operations, rarely if ever enhancing them. The fact that vaccines depress the immune system has been documented by a number of investigators. It is apparently this immunosuppressive action which largely accounts for their connection to cancer. Howenstine continues:

> *Cancer was a very rare illness in the 1890s. This evidence about immune system injury from vaccinating affords a plausible explanation for Dr. Clarke's finding that only vaccinated individuals got cancer. Some radical adverse change in health occurred in the early 1900s to permit cancer to explode and vaccinating appears to be the reason.*

Chapter 9
The Great Fraud

A vast fraud has been perpetrated upon the Western public. Lies have been told merely to promote certain agendas. Fear tactics have been used. For instance, consider the pro-immunization Web site, All About Moms. It merely perpetuates fear, particularly regarding the diseases of vaccinations. The entire approach is to create fear. This is in order to maintain the 'need' for vaccinations. There are a number of statements made on this Web site, which are adamant, that is biased. To quote the editors:

> *Immunization is the single most important way parents can protect their children against serious diseases. Children who have not been immunized are at a far greater risk of becoming infected with serious diseases (compared to who?). For example, a recent study showed that children who had not received the measles vaccine were 35 times more likely to get the disease...There are no effective alternatives to immunization for protection against serious and sometimes deadly infectious diseases.**

---

*This is a less-than-honest appraisal. For instance, P73 oregano oil, a potent germicidal spice oil, destroys deadly germs, such as the typical viruses for which vaccines are administered.

While breast-feeding can help to prevent some diseases among babies, it is not effective in preventing serious diseases that immunizations do.

Notice the emphasis on words such as serious, protection, deadly, etc. There is definite fear-mongering in these statements. Yet, the claim that measles is serious is misleading, since it is rarely disfiguring or fatal. Rather, cancer, lymphoma, retardation, diabetes and autism are serious, all of which are caused by vaccines. Even more significant are the statements that there are no other options for parents: 'only vaccines work.' This is an utter fabrication, a truly slanted statement. This is because a wide range of natural substances have been shown to destroy harmful pathogens as well as prevent infections by them. Furthermore, major improvements in diet as well as the appropriate nutritional supplements also are protective. What's more, contrary to the drug company's claim healthy breast-feeding, in fact, significantly reduces the incidence of the vaccine diseases and in some instances prevents them entirely.

The editors continue with a description of diseases which is revealing, describing virtually every disease for which children are vaccinated, many of which are largely extinct:

Diphtheria...can cause paralysis, breathing and heart problems, and death.

Tetanus...can cause muscle spasms, breathing and heart problems, and death.

Whooping cough...causes very long spells of coughing that make it hard for a child to eat, drink, or even breathe. Pertussis can cause lung problems, seizures, brain damage and death.

Hepatitis B (which is rare in children)...can cause liver damage, liver cancer and death.

Measles...can lead to hearing loss, pneumonia, brain damage, and even death.

Mumps...can lead to hearing loss, meningitis (inflammation of the brain and spinal cord) and brain damage.

Rubella...Pregnant women can lose their babies, or have babies with severe birth defects...

Polio causes fever and may progress to meningitis and/or lifelong paralysis. Polio can be fatal.

Chickenpox...can lead to serious complications such as inflammation of the brain and pneumonia, and rarely "flesh-eating" bacterial infection or death...as well as birth defects and infant death.

The fear-mongering is obvious. No mention is made regarding what causes such diseases. Nor are any preventive measures advised. Any parent who reads this would obviously feel compelled to pursue the recommended therapy. The editors close with the comment:

Immunizations are extremely safe and getting safer and more effective all the time as a result of medical research and ongoing review by doctors, researchers, and public health officials. Immunizations are given to keep healthy children well, so they are held to the highest safety standards. The number of immunizations has increased because we are now able to safely protect children from more serious diseases than ever before.

In contrast, it was J. Anthony Morris, M.D., former Chief of Vaccine Control at the FDA, who reported that vaccines, particularly the flu vaccine, fail to work and the pharmaceutical companies are well aware of it. He also reported that the flu vaccine increases the growth of cancerous tumors.

A review by public health officials at a government office, that is FDA officials, is no substitute for scientific investigation. The fact is the science demonstrates obvious toxicity due to vaccinations. No organ is immune from the devastation. As stated previously MD Anderson confirms that numerous cancers are caused by vaccinations, particularly lymphatic cancers. According to the *Journal of Pediatric Endocrinology* childhood diabetes is directly related to vaccinations. Finland's Dr. J. Classen has demonstrated that as many as 80% of all children with diabetes, that is Type 1 diabetics, have the disease as the result of vaccinations. Howenstine notes that in New Zealand after the introduction of an aggressive hepatitis B vaccination campaign the incidence of Type 1 diabetes rose some 60%. The fact is this vaccine is the primary cause of the sudden development of childhood diabetes. Is this synonymous with safety? The fact is the All About Moms site is riddled with lies. Rather, the site is an All About Convincing Moms to vaccinate.

The claim for safety on this drug company-sponsored site is highly specious. It is the PDR itself, a drug company publication which makes the dire toxicity of vaccines evident. Regarding one childhood vaccination alone, the DPT, it lists dozens of ominous side effects, including seizures, sudden death, shock, allergic reactions, convulsions, asthma reactions, infantile spasms, inflammation of the brain, inflammation of the spinal cord, paralysis, hives, swelling of the brain, and severe rash. Why would anyone allow such a substance to be injected in children, a known biological killer?

It was investigators in the Los Angeles County Coroner's Office, who confirmed the danger of this vaccine, fully correlating the DPT as a cause of sudden infant death syndrome. They discovered that dozens of infants died within a week of receiving the shot, some within the day. Tim O'Shea notes in his book, *The Sanctity of Human Blood*, an even more significant finding. This relates to a rash of infant deaths, all in a single state, Tennessee. Here, some 200 infants died suddenly, that is within 24 hours, after receiving the vaccination. No other cause for death could be found.

The MMR is equally fraught with dangers. It has been associated with an entire panorama of side effects, including muscle paralysis, palsies, retardation, blood clots, strokes, meningitis, Reye's syndrome, seizures, shock, sudden death, inflammation of the brain (encephalitis), joint inflammation, spinal cord damage, and diabetes. O'Shea further notes that such side effects fully prove the fraudulent nature of the claims for safety, since the very reason for giving the MMR is supposedly to prevent encephalitis as a complication of measles and/or mumps. How could a cause for such diseases also be the cure? Again, the aforementioned symptoms include both encephalitis and meningitis. What's more, if vaccinations are safe, why would the U. S. government exempt vaccine makers from lawsuits in the event of adverse reactions? The fact is the people who write such laws hold stock in these companies, even sitting on the Board of Directors. The fact is the government is well aware that vaccinations are a primary cause of death. To reiterate the Web site's position:

> *Immunizations are given to keep healthy children well, so they are held to the highest safety standards...*

Yet, it was the FDA itself which was forced in 2004 to condemn some 52 million doses of flu vaccine due to vast contamination. Throughout the Western world numerous vaccine makers have been essentially quarantined from further manufacturing until contamination issues are resolved. Wyeth alone has been cited by regulators dozens of times for manufacturing defects, primarily microbial contamination.

What high standards? Court records prove that Wyeth-Lederle, the maker of the modern polio vaccine, lied about quality control. For decades the company insisted it no longer used potentially contaminated monkeys, Rhesus macaques, as a source of organs for cell culture. This is the very monkey notoriously infected with SV40. Yet, all along the company was using the condemned species, fully risking human contamination. Further probing revealed that the FDA took the company at its word, never investigating the facilities to confirm compliance. The monkeys were continually used, putting all vaccine takers at risk for infection by a virus that is perhaps the most potent cause of cancer known.

Lederle was originally owned by American Cyanamid, a vast chemical/industrial conglomerate. Evidence of complicity by the company is found in the statements of Dr. John Martin, Professor of Pathology at the University of Southern California, who during the late 1970s worked as a virologist at the FDA. His job was to protect the public from any potential vaccine-induced contamination, since it was well known that vaccines by nature are contaminated. Well after concerns of contamination had been minimized Martin found that even as late as 1980 vaccine batches were seriously tainted. He discovered the existence of unknown germs in the lots, which were alive and infective and which could, thus, cause diseases unknown. Approaching his supervisors he warned them of this problem and was told to "discontinue his work as it was outside the scope of testing required for polio vaccine." Howenstine notes:

> Later, Dr. Martin learned that all eleven of the African green monkeys used to grow the Lederle polio virus...had grown simian cytomegalovirus from kidney cell cultures. Lederle was aware of this viral contamination...The (FDA) decided not to pursue the matter, so production of infected polio vaccine continued.

This is the supposedly trustworthy regulation that is proclaimed. It is nothing other than fraud. The government knew the vaccines were infected, and it did nothing. Despite this, pharmaceutical company propaganda proclaims that vaccines are safe, yet these companies provide no proof for their claims. They make innumerable broad statements for safety, as if any who dispute it are radicals—as if the mere dispute of this claim is a crime. Yet, it is the vaccine makers and their progenitors that are the criminals—remember the words of Anthony J. Morris, M.D., 'they know they are worthless, yet they sell them regardless.' This is a compelling statement from one of the world's top officials, the FDA's former Chief of Virology.

This is no attempt to radicalize anyone or create an "anti-government" approach. Rather, it is a revelation of the dangers inherent in man-made serums, admitted by top government authorities. It is a means to give people information, so they can protect themselves. Serums, that is inoculations, are derived from animal matter, including animal organs, secretions, and blood. Such substances are inherently contaminated. What's more, inherently, they are disease-causing.

For his statements Morris was fired, and his records were destroyed, burnt into oblivion. The fact is as the FDA is fully aware the making of vaccines fails to be a science and, rather, is a "sloppy and dangerous" practice. Infection of the batches by potentially destructive, in fact, carcinogenic, germs is a "huge unsolved current problem for all vaccine manufacturing." Thus, it would appear that the vaccine companies have no regard for human life. It's even reasonable to presume that they are even involved in a conspiracy against humans. This is confirmed by a paper published by the hierarchy of Rome, the so-called Club of Rome, which proclaims that there are too many humans on the Earth. This Club has deemed that the global population must be reduced by some 10%, apparently, by any means possible. Vaccines cause disease, despair and death. Apparently, there is a vicious purpose in their administration. Obviously, this Club has forgotten the dictates of their original scriptures that are its namesake, that is never purposely and maliciously take a human life, the life that the almighty creator has deemed sacred. Howenstine continues:

> ...what could be a more diabolically clever way to eliminate people than to inject them with a cancer-causing vaccine? The person receiving the injection would never suspect that the vaccine taken 10 to 15 years earlier had caused the cancer to appear.

Even vaccine proponents have registered warnings. It was Jonas Salk, M.D., the originator of the Salk polio vaccine, who stated that regarding live viral vaccines in each instance they may "produce the disease it intended to prevent. The live virus against measles and mumps may produce such side effects as encephalitis (a common cause of brain damage, which can be fatal)." In other words, vaccines are a dangerous procedure, a kind of medicine with potentially fatal consequences. Thus, it becomes clear that if possible vaccinations should be avoided.

It was Robert Mendelsohn, M.D., whose landmark book, *How to Raise a Healthy Child in Spite of Your Doctor*, made clear the true nature of vaccinations. As a pediatrician in his vast medical experience he observed a wide range of diseases actually caused by this therapy. He said that modern vaccinations are the "greatest threat" to a child's health, noting that "There is no convincing scientific evidence that mass inoculations can be credited with eliminating any childhood disease." What an incredible statement it is, by an internationally renowned pediatrician, that all modern vaccines are valueless. After many years of research and treating patients this was Mendelsohn's personal assessment. What's more, he stated, "There are significant risks associated with every immunization." This too is a compelling observation, again based upon personal experience. This means that the greater the number of injections there are the greater is the risk for long-term or acute damage. Finally, he queries, "Have we traded mumps and measles for cancer and leukemia?" Then, he advises that parents, as well as adults, should "reject all immunizations." While in his late 60s Dr. Mendelsohn died under suspicious circumstances.

The link of modern vaccines to cancers is difficult to dismiss. It was Ted Koren in his book, *Childhood Vaccines*, who demonstrated it. He notes that between 1960 and 1980 there was an immense increase in North America of childhood cancers, the very era when vaccines were doubled. The fact is these two decades were the era of the mandatory vaccine. Even the CDC in a 1989 report documents the toxic effects of vaccines upon the immune system, notably, the measles vaccine, which it reported causes an "immune suppression which contributes to an increased susceptibility to other infections." In other words, instead of boosting or improving immunity vaccines diminish it. Thus, the body is highly vulnerable to tumor growth. What's more, this damage may be regarded as permanent, although to a degree some function can be recovered (see Appendix A).

Risky business

Jonas Salk was in a rush. Yet, this is true of most vaccine makers. The whole process of vaccine manufacture is "slip-shod." Shortcuts are taken, which put the population at risk. Independent scientific studies are rarely if ever performed.

When Salk promoted his vaccine, researchers had to rely upon *his* science and *his* procedures. No independent confirmation was performed. What's more, what little confirmation which was performed was merely done by reviewing his findings. Furthermore, the reviewer, Dr. Franklin, was Salk's professor as well as colleague.

> *Incredibly, Franklin was the sole researcher selected to review and ultimately approve Salk's work. Said Sarah Riedman in her propaganda-riddled, "Shots Without Guns: The Story of Vaccination":*

> *...despite his fondness for his former student, he could be trusted to give impartial judgement.*

Can anyone truly believe that this was an impartial jury? The fact is both Francis and Salk were under the pay of the Foundation for Infantile Paralysis, today's March of Dimes, and, thus, it was in both their interests for the vaccination to be approved. Both were in a 'rush' to gain acceptance. Both had a vested interest in the approval of a mass vaccination plan, and both stood to lose from the lack of approval. Thus, the entire process was from the outset tainted. Even before the vaccine was approved vaccine companies had produced millions of vials. There was too much at stake for a failure to approve. The entire process was in a rush mode. Disasters could be expected, and this is precisely what occurred. Riedman describes the scenario as follows:

> *Within a few days after the announcement that the Salk polio vaccine was "safe, potent, effective," children trooped in line to receive the first shots of vaccine...Within a week four million doses had been shipped to health officers to build up the defenses against the anticipated summer attack of polio. But just*

as it seemed that the new vaccine was closing in on polio, there was a tragic setback in the campaign.

At the end of April came the alarming news that polio had developed in a number of children who had been inoculated. The vaccine was traced...to one firm... Something had gone wrong! Further distribution from the particular drug company was stopped...Eleven persons had died and 200 had developed polio.

Despite this Riedman proclaims in her book the program a success. How could it be a success, to brutalize, maim, and kill others? This was mere marketing hype to establish the 'credibility' of the organization. There was no basis for such a claim. As her only evidence she quotes spotty breakouts of polio, claiming that in these outbreaks the vaccinated were protected to a greater degree than the people who failed to get vaccinated. She fails to consider, however, the fact that numerous people who failed to get vaccinated developed the disease as a result of being exposed to the vaccinated. The fact is of the two hundred cases of polio resulting shortly after the introduction of the vaccine some 40% were unvaccinated family members, who got the disease from vaccinated children.

Soon after it was instituted the vaccine killed dozens of people. Yet, Riedman would have her readers believe that the polio vaccine's progenitors, Salk and Sabin, were national heros. This was a 'professional' cover-up. The consequences of their 'discovery' was an merciless global cancer epidemic.

Yet, while the number of deaths may seem low the fact is such individuals were in perfect health until they were vaccinated. What's more, some 200 others developed permanent paralysis as a result of the vaccination, ruining their lives. What a debacle it was: hundreds of human lives destroyed, all as a result of the aggressive rush to market of an unproven therapy. Yet, this was only the reported cases. There were obviously many others, thousands, perhaps, tens of thousands more, whose plight will never be known. What's more, these are only the victims of the acute damage occurring shortly after the introduction of the vaccine. Surely, over the course of some seven years, when the Sabin and Salk vaccines were in primary use, there were uncountable others who were also harmed, whose representations will never be known. Then, there are the other countless victims, who were/are chronically damaged—who were/are infected by contaminants unknown as well as SV40. The number of individuals who were/are permanently traumatized as a result of these vaccines is beyond measure, but the fact is it numbers in the tens of millions.

The Sabin vaccine, which was delivered through sugary syrups and sugar cubes, was also widely distributed. It was extensively tested in Russia (that is the former Soviet Union), Czechoslovakia, Mexico, and Poland. All the recipients in such regions were infected with SV40.

The Salk/Sabin vaccine fiasco is no minor medical mishap. The fact is it is the greatest medical catastrophe of all time. This is because, as has been documented throughout this book, the vaccine is directly related to the catastrophe which thwarts all humanity: the modern cancer epidemic. So much for the dictum, "safe, potent, effective."

The Sabin-invented sugar cube was also rushed to market. Sabin simply concocted the idea of using the sugar cube to distribute it. In fact, this was a dangerous, ill-conceived method, since sugar increases the virulence of the virus. It is well known that outbreaks of polio coincided with the increase in sugar consumption. Yet perhaps more diabolically, like the Salk vaccine, it was merely decided that this was the most convenient method: no independent research was performed to prove safety or efficacy. The fact is the monkey serum-tainted sugar cube was a most grotesque joke against humankind.

By 1963 some 70 million Americans, in addition to millions of others globally, received the vaccine. Totals vary, but it is estimated that some 100 million North Americans were ultimately directly infected with SV40 through contaminated Salk and Sabin vaccines. Surely, those receiving the live virus-based sugar cube or sugary syrup gained the greatest dose of this agent.

Regarding the polio vaccine the Salk Papers, published after this researcher's death, prove the vast degree of corruption. These papers are found at the University of California, San Diego, in the University Library. The March of Dimes was heavily involved in Salk's career, largely funding his research.

This organization was dependent upon public funds for its agenda, which, originally, was largely based upon a mass vaccination plan. It also relied upon a real or perceived polio cure to maintain donations. Internal memos prove that without creating a public image of the development of such a cure, there was concern that the organization would collapse. Thus, the March of Dimes orchestrated a massive push to meet its goals. A panic was purposely created, which caused a public clamoring for the vaccine. A similar approach is applied for today's vaccines. Public pressure became unbearable; legislators joined the foray. Incredibly, rather than the medical profession it was the lay public, as well as the politicians, who set the agenda for medical practice. While well trained to do so these sources dictated the pressures that led to the mass vaccination program.

In the 1960s Salk created the Salk Institute. This was only possible because of public donations, since "A substantial amount of the start-up funds came from the National Foundation-March of Dimes." Here, Salk continued to research and develop new vaccines. For his original vaccine, again, the March of Dimes was the funding source. The organization itself was founded by President Franklin Roosevelt, himself a victim of polio. He contracted it as an adult, most likely as a result of exposure to sewage-tainted water while vacationing. The president of the foundation, Basil O'Conner, was Roosevelt's former law partner. This demonstrates a conflict of interest. Thus, the entire project was suspect from its inception. This is, essentially, an example of the government practicing medicine, rather, of lawyers doing so.

Salk's research was fully dependent upon government funds, and such monies were derived, incredibly, from public donations. Yet, it was this very public who suffered harm from its own generosity. In the process of creating the vaccine, experimenting with it, and achieving its approval the (March of Dimes) was "Deeply involved..." This again proves that the government was mandating policy in an area in which it was unschooled, that is the prevention and cure of disease.

Thus, the polio vaccine was based to a greater extent upon government policy than any proven need. Polio was in a steep decline. Why institute an expensive government-mandated treatment for a disease that was plummeting in incidence? If there was a need for such intervention, why not select a disease that was a major killer: high blood pressure, heart disease, diabetes, or cancer? To select a disease that was exponentially declining in incidence? It makes no medical sense. Then, why should it? Rather than medical scientists it was orchestrated by the government.

Government-enforced health care can only lead to catastrophes, particularly when it is instituted by untrained individuals. Now, due to this ill-conceived plan millions suffer, while untold other thousands have prematurely died. This fails to include those primary victims who shortly after being vaccinated died from the vaccinations.

There is no proof that the injection of proteins and unknown contaminants of monkey kidney/testicular tissue into humans is safe. The fact is it would be expected that the injection of such matter would be dangerous. What's more, there is no proof that any vaccine is sterile. Rather, common sense would dictate that such solutions, derived from diseased caged animals, would be widely infected. Obviously, the ingestion or injection of such a contaminated solution would create a vast degree of pathology. All a person would have to do is simply look at the various monkeys used for the research. It would readily conclude that their tissues should never be safely injected nor ingested—in any form, including a chemically neutralized one—into a human. What's more, consider formaldehyde, a known carcinogen and a cause of allergic and chemical toxicity. Could this by any standard be deemed safe for human injection, particularly the injection into infants and children? Vaccine companies routinely do this, and the government encourages it. Yet, as a result of vaccine reactions every year numerous babies die. Such a thinking is truly bizarre, yet, scientists rarely if ever consider such consequences.

As demonstrated by British investigators the March of Dimes protocol, that is the aggressive promotion of the Salk and Sabin vaccines, was a catastrophe. It led in many regions of the United States to an increase in the incidence of polio. It caused a wide range of diseases unknown. It is directly connected to a variety of cancers, and this connection is indisputable. It appears to be the major man-made factor in the rising incidence of blood and lymphatic cancer, particularly the various types of lymphomas. Incredibly, the latter disease is a man-made disaster. Untold thousands of individuals, innocent unwitting victims, have died as a consequence of this policy, many a gruesome death. How could it also possibly be regarded as beneficial? If this is the gold-standard of what modern medicine has to offer, its main success—the fact is this is incredible. Yet, it is natural medicines that are offering the cure for this catastrophe. This is because edible wild oregano (the Oreganol P73) has directly destroyed all viruses against which it has been tested, including SV40. Man destroys himself and, then, the great divine being provides the cure. This is a testimony for the fact that humans must rely upon almighty God—the natural powers—rather than the synthetic 'god' of medicine.

The March of Dimes falsely promoted itself as the savior of humankind, when in fact it was its destroyer. It promoted itself as truly humanitarian. People trusted in this and donated profusely. This led to the outgrowth of a number of other supposedly humanitarian organizations, which also claimed as their agendas the conquest of 'incurable' diseases such as multiple sclerosis, cystic fibrosis, and muscular dystrophy. It is interesting to note that a high incidence of multiple sclerosis, as well as muscular dystrophy, is found only in populations which are heavily vaccinated. How convenient: create the disease and, then, make the claim for its cure in order to garner greater donations.

There is always the counter-claim, that is for lives saved. It is the claim that with such vaccines the disasters are overshadowed by the benefit: that the loss or harm to the few is "overshadowed by the thousands of people who have remained alive and unparalyzed...had they not taken the shots." This is mere speculation. No one can claim this as a certainty. Perhaps it is true, but perhaps this is wishful thinking—perhaps mere propaganda. The fact is Klein, who was in fact favorable to the vaccine, created a kind of supposition, which requires careful analysis to demonstrate its fallacy:

The Salk vaccine was far from perfect. The cases dropped sharply from 1954 on, but there were some 2000 reported cases in 1959. People died from receiving improperly prepared vaccine...

Is this anything other than a catastrophe of the greatest extreme? The very medicine which is supposed to halt an epidemic, to protect the public from harm, in fact, causes harm? Polio was already on the decline. Improvements in sanitation resulted in that. There was no way to prove, for a steadily declining disease, that the vaccine was responsible. The incidence of this disease had so precipitously declined that proof of a cure through vaccination was now impossible. Rather, it would appear that the introduction of the vaccine led to an outbreak: in 1959. This is because the 2000 new cases which then occurred represented an unexplainable spike in the incidence. As further proof of the corrupt nature of this program Klein continues:

A great price was paid of the vaccines of the 1950s and 1960s...Scientific endeavor was frequently reduced to the level of merchandising, and the alleged objectivity of scientists was severely strained in the intensity of competition. It was a vivid reminder that science had become big business...The commercialization of science started long before the polio-vaccine spectacle. Ever since governments and all varieties of entrepreneurs realized that useful products could result from the application of (science) pressure has been exerted on scientists to spend more time on designing things...

In other words, rather than careful science profits were the priority. This led directly to an epidemic that Westerners now endure: the contamination of the human body with various simian and other animal viruses, known to cause cancer.

Regarding public donations the polio campaign was a success. Rather than for research most of the money collected directly from the public was used for marketing. It was the public who paid for the polio vaccination. They were engaged by clever marketing to 'give generously.' What they failed to realize was that they paid for their own horror. The more they gave the more sophisticated the marketing became. The same technique was utilized by its followers, including the various cancer foundations heavily promoted today.

Following World War II the U.S. government increasingly played a role in medical research. Organizations such as the American Cancer Society developed, which successfully solicited money from the public. There was no accounting for how this money was used. Then, in 1971 Nixon declared a war on cancer. Willingly or not, every American taxpayer became a contributor. All such money was squandered primarily on pharmaceutical research as well as to maintain the self-serving agendas of the foundations. At the government's behest billions of dollars were poured into supposed research. Yet, not the slightest cure has been produced. Nor were the true causes for cancer discovered. Nor was there any accountability for how the money was spent. This is despite the fact that virtually the entire modern cancer epidemic was caused by the organization. Again, it used the peoples' own money to, incredibly, infect them. This is the consequence of public generosity. The fact is it is a crime against humanity, and the average person is the victim.

Cancer is caused by viral infections. It may also be caused by bacterial and fungal infections. The epidemic now afflicting Westerners coincides with the increase in vaccine use. Several early American physicians, including Bush, noted that prior to vaccinations cancer was rare. Clearly, such physicians knew that vaccinations were cancer-causing.

Since they are made from animal components by nature vaccines are contaminated. This is why harsh chemicals, as well as irradiation, are used to decontaminate them. Yet, this is impossible to do. There is always the risk that some components of the contamination—some potentially invasive germs or germ elements—remain, that is biologically active. There can be no possible benefit from the ingestion/injection of such agents. Thus, vaccines are disease-promoting.

With their therapies drug companies are poisoning the masses. Vaccines cause toxic fulminant reactions in the blood and internal organs. How else could they be responsible for such extreme consequences such as attention deficit, autism, multiple sclerosis, paralysis, muscular degeneration, autoimmune disorders, ulcerative colitis, Crohn's disease, ankylosing spondylitis, pericarditis, lupus, immune system disorders, juvenile arthritis, diabetes, and cancer.

Vaccines are a kind of drug. Like drugs they function by suppressing the symptoms. They fail to cure the disease. Rather, they cause disease. The fact is there are entire diseases due to vaccinations. These include diseases which had previously been unknown. Such diseases include autism, attention deficit syndrome, mesothelioma, scleroderma, ankylosing spondylitis, and certain types of brain and blood cancers. The aforementioned are caused virtually exclusively by vaccinations. Regarding the polio vaccine it specifically causes mesothelioma, choroid plexus brain tumors, and non-Hodgkin's lymphoma. This proves that vaccines cause a variety of devastating diseases.

The public placed its trust in the system, and this system failed them. Now millions of people are faced with a catastrophe of an unprecedented degree: vast chronic illnesses, which are destroying the fabric of civilization and are prematurely taking uncountable human lives.

Polio: a disease of sanitation?

These catastrophes could have been prevented. When the polio vaccines were being given, this disease was declining significantly. Without the vaccine, eventually, the disease would have died out. In the Western world running water became 'nationalized,' as did proper sewage and garbage disposal. As these procedures became more thoroughly established the incidence of diseases of sanitation, including polio, cholera, diphtheria, and typhoid fever, exponentially declined. There was no need for the vaccine. The fact is when it was introduced, there was no polio epidemic. Again, the polio virus is a fecal pathogen, largely a contaminant from open sewer wastes. The connection of poor sanitation is readily described by Roland H. Berg, in his book, the *Challenge of Polio*. It was Berg who revealed early studies proving the entire epidemic as due to defects in cleanliness and sanitation. Says Berg regarding a polio outbreak in North Carolina (1944):

> *There was a score of tasks for these doctors to perform here in the backwoods section of North Carolina. But one thing they decided not to overlook was the role of flies in carrying and spreading (polio). To do this they set up a novel experiment (with bananas). (They)...selected a home where a young child had been taken ill with (polio). In the patient's home the bananas were peeled and sliced into open dishes. After sprinkling some sugar on the top they placed dishes of sliced bananas on the kitchen table and warned the family not to touch the bait... For two days the bananas remained on the kitchen table with flies constantly buzzing around and settling on the food. When the investigator had decided that the food had been contaminated as much as possible, they packed the dish of sliced bananas, freezing it...for shipment to the*

lab...The (doctors) fed the bananas to two chimpanzees...Immediately, tests of the feces...were begun. Within a short time the doctors were amazed by the discovery that the bowel eliminations...were loaded with the virus...

This was absolute proof that polio is a disease of poor sanitation. It was a filth disease, which could easily be eradicated through modernization. True, the wealthier people were contracting it, but this was to a degree due to the excessive incidence of tonsillectomy, again combined with hygienic deficiencies such as swimming in contaminated water. Yet, here too by merely creating a high attention to hygiene and public health, plus solid nutrition, the disease was preventable. What's more, outbreaks of polio were associated with poor nutrition. The fact is these outbreaks were directly coincident with the increase in intake of processed foods, particularly refined sugar. People who rarely ate such foods seemed immune.

Regarding the sliced banana technique the mechanism of the spread of polio was elucidated by these researchers. They discovered that while the chimpanzees remained healthy despite eating the polio-tainted food, when their feces were injected into uninfected animals they developed the disease. This is a disconcerting finding, that is that poor hygiene may spread the disease from a 'healthy' carrier to an innocent uninfected individual. The conclusion of the researchers was, therefore, compelling: that poor hygiene causing infection orally is the primary cause of polio. In other words, dirty hands and food, soil with fecal matter or general filth are the ready sources of its spread. Recall in the backwoods of North Carolina even the idea of washing, as well as bathing, was unknown, let alone cleansing the hands, for instance, after defecating. The fact is in such regions there was little if any running water. What's more, outhouses were common. Thus, rather than vaccination the cure was in upgrading living standards. In general in a region where there is normal sanitation and where there is full attention to hygiene, as well as good nutrition, outbreaks of this disease are eliminated.

In the 1930s and 1940s there were occasional outbreaks of polio, particularly in 'backward' regions, that is areas where sanitation systems had not been fully established. In other words, in the more primitive regions of the United States 'sewage still ran in the streets.' Berg quotes an illustrative case:

> ...(regarding) swimming in polluted (water), scientific research has piled up a wealth of...evidence...in a small town in Perrysburg, Ohio which suffered an outbreak of polio in the summer of 1944. Perrysburg is a community of only 3500 persons, and the occurrence of eleven cases...was a catastrophe. The townspeople were in a state of panic and fear.

Yet, what people failed to realize was that there was no need for panic and despair. This is because this disease could be eradicated without draconian measures and/or mass vaccinations. This is because polio is largely a disease of sanitation. In his analysis of further war-time polio outbreaks Berg described further cases, which are revealing. These outbreaks occurred in the United States before sanitation systems were fully in place. According to Berg:

> Doctors...surveyed the town, and discovered that a majority of the patients lived in homes bordering a creek that ran though the settlement. The scientists decided to make a search for the virus in the waters of that muddy stream. Their suspicions....were strengthened when the local chief of police told them that he knew of several children who had contracted (polio) after wading and swimming in the creek.

"Some of them," he said, "had upset stomachs after swimming in the water." There was evidence also that the stream was being polluted at a number of places by...sewage.

After collecting many samples of creek water the scientists left Perrysburg and returned to the laboratory to begin the arduous work of proving the presence of the virus...The first animals...died shortly after inoculation with the samples (in other words, there was no way to tell if these animals would contract polio; they died too quickly). The second animals (also quickly) died...but doggedly the scientists continued with the inoculations into other rats. Finally their efforts were reared. The seventh series (of injected rats) showed symptoms...To confirm their results they removed the spinal cord and brains of the dead rats and injected an emulsion of this into monkeys. When the monkeys became sick and paralyzed with polio the research work was complete. The polio scientists had proved that the creek water contained the virus...

Further proof for the sanitation connection is the fact that in the 1940s the majority of outbreaks occurred in the summer, when festering heat increased the risks for the spread in sewage-tainted regions. The role of flies in spreading the disease is also confirmed by the summer outbreaks. During that era the country was attending to war, not the improvement of the nation's infrastructure. Berg continues:

In the summer of 1941 there occurred what was to be known as the Tragedy at Akron. This became one of the greatest opportunities of medical sleuthing in the recorded history of polio research. A tragedy-stricken home in Akron became the mecca of polio scientists...to seek out the reasons for the crippler's visitation.

The city of Akron during the summer of 1941 had been relatively free of (polio). A few cases occurred sporadically...but the number was not alarming. There was no evidence of a present or impending epidemic...yet, in that peaceful midwestern city polio was to engulf a typically American family, striking five of the family's six children and killing three of them. The K family was old-fashioned in its size—father, mother, and six children—ranging from an eleven-year-old boy to a two-and-one-half-year-old boy. Suddenly and mysteriously (polio) struck at this little home. Five of the six children developed the disease. In a few days the oldest children were dead; the other two survived, but (were crippled) for the rest of their lives.

Never before in the history of polio had there occurred such a tragedy. Multiple cases in one family had been known but never to the extent experienced by the K family. It immediately became the center of interest of all those scientific workers engaged in tracking down the mysterious virus.

A score of workers invaded the...home. Finally after months of questioning and study the complete story unfolded...On July 1, the mother, father and the four oldest children visited an aunt who had a little cottage on Dollar Lake, a resort near Akron. The other two children were left during this time with another aunt (whose son) was operated on and his tonsils were removed. (This son)...for about a week was mildly ill and then recovered...

...the five oldest children were taken to a local physician for a general examination. The doctor suggested that all five of them have their tonsils

removed...The day before the operations...three of the oldest children went picnicking and fishing with some of their friends at a nearby pond. It was a dirty pool filled with rushes and stagnant water. However, this didn't deter the children...and they ate their sandwiches on the bank, fished and waded in the water.

The next day all five of the oldest children were brought to the hospital to have their tonsils and adenoids removed. In addition, the four oldest had several teeth extracted. *The operations were done under (general) anesthesia...After spending the afternoon in the hospital the children were taken home.

During the next few days the children remained comparatively quiet although they did visit with some of the neighborhood children, and went wading again...Six days after their operation the five children were all taken to the physicians who examined their throats and considered their condition satisfactory. Three days later one of the K children, the seven-year-old who had had his tonsils removed, complained of not feeling well. He was listless and refused to eat...(and then developed) abdominal pains and...vomiting...In addition, two of the other children began complaining of vague pains.

The illness progressed rapidly and within twenty-four hours four of the children had developed definite signs of paralysis...and the children were admitted with the diagnosis of (polio). Two days after their admission...three of the children were dead. (Yet,

---

* This is critical, since such extractions can spread the virus into the brain and spinal cord, creating a fatal infection. The extractions themselves can spread germs into the bloodstream, suppressing the immune response.

incredibly,)...the youngest child who had not been operated on, and the mother and father remained perfectly well.

This is an incredible testimony. The fact is all the cases of polio occurred in children who underwent tonsillectomy, and in some cases tooth extraction, while those who retained their tonsils were protected. The higher risk for polio coincides directly with the increase in the use of these procedures. There is further compelling proof. Of all countries the United States was the main focus of polio outbreaks, which occurred largely in the summer. Of course, this is when children were available to "get their tonsils out." Plus, it was in the United States where the highest number of these procedures were performed. Perhaps all along in the United States rather than a brutal act of nature polio was a man-made disease, to a degree perpetrated by the medical profession. Tonsillectomy was one such brutal therapy which caused the onset and spread of this disease.

Obviously, the tonsils play a vast role in protecting the body from such invaders. The fact is even though the aforementioned children had waded in dirty water it is unlikely that they would have developed this disease and/or died if their tonsils and adenoids would have been intact, since these organs would have protected them from the illness. Thus, with all the panic and pandemonium and, therefore, the future call for the vaccine, there was a failure to analyze the possible causes for this epidemic, for instance, the destructive action upon the body of tonsillectomy. What's more, as polio, especially in teenagers and adults, was regarded as a "rich-man's disease," it makes sense that it would be related to this newfangled operation. The fact is the vast majority of tonsillectomies were done on the middle and upper class.

The connection is clear. Since polio is an intestinal virus, which is found throughout the mucous membranes, the violent removal of these glands spread the disease. The fact is residues of this virus are known to exist within the tonsils and adenoids, and as the aforementioned cases demonstrate, surgically treated children became readily infected. What's more, if such children naturally had the virus in their intestines, then, the removal of the highly protective tonsils, which guard the most critical regions of the body—the oral and upper nasal cavities and their connection to the brain, left the individuals vulnerable. No longer did they have their miraculously powerful lymph organs intact, so strategically, in fact, divinely, placed near the potentially vulnerable regions, that is near the entrances to the brain, to protect them from viral invasion. Most likely, during surgery the virus was liberated from the tonsillar or adenoid tissues, where it readily hides, and, now that there was no lymphatic protection, entered the brain. There could also have been regurgitation of intestinal material upwards, due to the effects on the bowel of anesthesia. Then, in an immune compromised environment it reproduced, causing infection.

Apparently, the original source (the aunt's son) became immune. However, the visitors acquired it and had no immunity. The infection developed in them and, then, due to the lack of the highly protective tonsils and adenoids, so strategically placed near the access areas to the brain, spread into the nervous system, killing two of the children. What's more, the procedure was unnecessary and was most likely advised for financial gain. Thus, the deaths of these children were doctor-induced and may not have been due exclusively to problems of sanitation. In this case the giving of the vaccine would have been of no consequence.

Berg reiterates the true source of these deaths as due to the surgical procedure:

> The virus was demonstrated to be present in many persons without clinical symptoms. Why then did it select the five K children for its vicious attack? There was one factor that was different. The five K children had

undergone adenoid and tonsil operation. This fact had greater weight when it was realized that the youngest, the two-and-one-half-year-old, had virus in his stool as well as the older brothers and sisters. But he was not operated on...and he was the only one...to escape...

True, it is possible that the children inoculated themselves with the virus through swimming and wading in filthy water. Or, they may have contracted it from their tonsillectomized cousin. Interestingly, the height of the polio epidemic coincided with the height of the use of this surgery. What's more, tonsillectomy is a surgery very close to the brian. Thus its role in causing neurological infection is obvious.

This proves a simple fact, that is the powerful immunity and versatility of children. As long as their immune systems were intact, no infection, and certainly no polio, developed. This demonstrates that with a healthy immunity, intact immune glands, the avoidance of draconian medical procedures, and proper sanitation there is no possibility of polio epidemics.

This documents a simple fact. Modern medical procedures cause various diseases. Rather than an act of God many such diseases are also due to negligence. The failure to properly cleanse the body, particularly the failure to attend to proper handwashing, is a primary cause of disease. Poor hygienic practices, for instance, the lack of thorough bathing, particularly after being exposed to filth, such as might occur from swimming in public waters or contaminated streams: all could lead to serious diseases, even death. It is these issues which must be first addressed, not a massive push for national vaccination.

For no good reason the tonsils and adenoids have been stripped from the bodies of untold millions of individuals. This has greatly increased the risks for various diseases, particularly cancer and neurological disorders. These organs exist for deliberate reasons. They are the body's immunological sentinels, guarding the gate of entry, the nasal cavity and mouth, from noxious substances and, particularly, from dangerous germs. The polio virus is a bowel virus. Without the protective actions of the tonsils and adenoids this virus could aggressively invade the tissues, including the brain and spinal cord. The fact is a review of the medical files during this era, the 1940s through 1960s, when tonsillectomy was popularized, reveals a significant number of complications, including sudden death: directly due to the surgery.

Incredibly, the surgeons largely created the polio epidemic. After childrens' immune systems were weakened due to the lack of lymphatic glands the medical system foisted the vaccine upon the public, claiming a cure. What a barbaric approach it was. Yet, it is also clearly a fraud, since polio was strictly in decline, this as a consequence of vast improvements in sanitation as well as the food supply. What's more, as polio was endemic, that is already within the intestines and mucous membranes, surgery simply furthered its spread. Furthermore, while polio is rare a wide range of polio-like conditions, which also cause paralysis, are prolific. The fact is Guillain Barré is essentially a 'modern' kind of polio, as is multiple sclerosis. Thus, polio has not been eradicated, rather, it has merely been re-named. Thus, rather than any vaccine-related cure paralytic diseases still exist.

Tonsillectomies increase the risks for a variety of other diseases, particularly immune deficiency disorders, chronic infections, and cancers. By systematically removing the tonsils from children and then vaccinating them with SV40-tainted vaccines surgeons greatly increased their risks for the development of cancer. Because of these two ill-conceived 'therapies' thousands of children have died from cancers. The same is true of adults, who readily develop cancers as a result of SV40 and tonsillectomy.

The human body is a magnificent creation. It is highly sophisticated and organized. If it is corrupted, disease will result. All efforts should be made to keep the body in its original state and to resist any attempts to disrupt and/or corrupt it. Surgery should only be performed in life-threatening disorders and when absolutely necessary. Their should be no exceptions to this rule.

The culling of Americans

SV40 infection has decimated much of the human race. How could anyone even remotely consider the injection of monkey blood/secretions into humans as safe? Did such researchers simply not care? Were they so enamored of themselves that they neglected all for mere material gain?

This animal pathogen is responsible for untold pain and agony—the unmerciful suffering of the human masses. Plus, it is responsible for the premature deaths of vast numbers of humans, too extensive to count. Even so, a reasonable estimate is that this ill-conceived project has harmed tens of millions, in fact, hundreds of millions, of individuals. The polio vaccine is a terror weapon, foisted upon the masses by arrogant scientists, who, rather than honoring human needs pursued their own wicked agenda. Remember, this program largely caused the cancer epidemic. That such scientists were arrogant and indifferent cannot be disputed. The fact is such individuals well knew that monkey pathogens are highly aggressive, capable of causing serious diseases.

The most dangerous of these vaccines was produced during the mid-1950s and early 1960s. This was when the SV40 epidemic was initiated. Who should be responsible for such a crime, where the health of millions of individuals have been devastated? Salk and Sabin were held as national heros. Is it heroic to kill the innocent? Is it the way of heros to slowly and methodically denude and corrupt the health of hundreds of millions of people, all under the guise of "saving" them? This fully demonstrates how bizarre, in fact, corrupt, modern medicine truly is.

Consider this: there would be no deaths from certain cancers—or the deaths would be exceedingly low—were it not for the polio vaccine. Since its inception those million or so cases of lymphoma; perhaps the majority of those cancers would never have appeared. Regarding brain cancers in children the majority are SV40-induced, although other similar viruses may play a role, including the notorious B monkey virus. Thus, instead of saving lives the polio vaccine caused death and destruction. This was a murderous campaign, and regarding this there can be no dispute. Yet, perhaps the most critical issue is the fact that almighty God made medicines, which are more effective than vaccines in preventing disease. Thus, there is no need to inject the body with contaminants. Injecting the germ does not cure the disease but, rather, it merely modifies how the body reacts to it. There are natural ways to deal with virtually any infection. There is no need to fear.

In epidemics there may be the rare need for vaccines. Yet, certain natural medicines, particularly oil of wild oregano, cold-pressed garlic oil, and wild cumin oil, are so powerful that they are far more reliable for protection than inoculations. What's more, while vaccines have caused epidemics, including the TB and SV40 epidemics, natural medicines have never caused any such gross harm.

Incredibly, the very substance which causes epidemics is also used to treat them? The cause cannot also be the treatment. This is a bizarre approach, which violates common sense. It cannot be that the injection of potentially lethal contaminants can create health. Surely, the polio vaccine debacle demonstrates that. To 'trade' a supposed reduction in the incidence of polio with a vast increase in cancer as well as litany of other diseases: is this the best that medicine can offer? Medical authorities boast about grandiose vaccination campaigns. The fact is the polio vaccine campaign alone largely created the cancer epidemic.

Rather than cause disease doctors are supposed to cure it. How could any researcher, any organization, perpetrate such an act: to inject contaminated monkey serum, or to give it orally, to the healthy population? This has caused a vast degree of harm, and the American and Canadian public are the primary victims. American citizens were the main focus of the mass polio vaccination plan. Children lined up and received their injection, syrup, and/or sugar cube. If such children moved to new regions and failed to have available their records, they received additional doses. Thus, it is no surprise that a minimum of 25% of all Americans have SV40 in their blood, while, incredibly, some 50% of all males have it in their sperm.

Yet, all such contamination was preventable. This is because there was foreknowledge of the destructive nature of the vaccine, even before it was given. As early as 1960 it was known that the oral polio sugar cube was tainted. Researchers had fully proven that many of the batches—if not all the batches—which were being prepared for public dissemination were infected. What's more, as demonstrated by Lear in *Recombinant DNA* researchers had categorically determined that the contaminants were carcinogenic and that it was likely that the recipients would develop cancer. Yet, as described by Lear the vaccines were administered regardless, with utter indifference to the consequences.

The vaccine itself had proven unreliable in rendering immunity to exposed subjects. According to Schaeffer's *Experimental Poliomyelitis* even after being fully vaccinated when exposed to airborne viruses some 90% of test subjects developed the infection. This study was done well before the vaccine was released. Thus, the vaccine failed to even achieve its purported claim.

Yet, perhaps most critically the polio vaccine was administered at a time when there was no polio epidemic. Then, since there was no benchmark to measure it against how could its efficacy be determined?

Even the direct consequences of the vaccine, that is sudden fatal or near-fatal reactions, were predictable. It quickly became evident that these supposed therapies killed and maimed people, and, yet, the authorities continued to administer them. Were such supposed experts intent upon destroying the human race—was their goal to cause unmerciful harm? Or, were they merely duped by the medical hype? Or, perhaps, did they deem themselves as if almighty? Yet, this demonstrates how truly barbaric is the modern medical approach and powerful it is, that is that the entire world can be convinced that a destroyer is a cure.

From the polio vaccine alone hundreds of thousands of people died prematurely. Untold other hundreds of thousands have suffered inordinately, for instance, with chronic wasting disease. It would appear that the human race, particularly the American public, is merely a guinea pig for the powerful chemical and drug cartel, which commits its devious acts at will. The fact is unless people resist such tyranny, shortly, such acts will result in the demise of the human race. No one will be able to resist: all will be forced to submit, that is to the powers-that-be. People need to resist such tyranny in every way possible, including speaking out against such crimes.

The Sabin/Salk vaccine was a crime against humanity. Yet, will the human race remain subdued as such high crimes continue? The individual must do all that is possible to halt such criminal acts on this earth. One way to do so is to refuse to use or buy such destructive elements. Regarding vaccines a political or religious exemption is sufficient. Or, a doctor's excuse can be prescribed advising against the use of the vaccine due to allergy or sensitivity. Legal documents can be drafted warning the responsible parties, that is the doctors, nurses, hospital staff, and school board members, for the need for indemnification. In other words, if any such persons attempt to mandate the vaccine then they must sign a waver requiring that they take responsibility for any damages. If the vaccine causes harm, for instance, autism, multiple sclerosis, or cancer, then they are held responsible. Regarding the religious exemption see Appendix B.

To American society in particular vaccines have caused immeasurable damage. Here, the decline in human health has greatly affected productivity. If a person is sick, how can he/she function efficiently? The fact is as a result of damage from SV40 some individuals are fully dysfunctional. Thus, they are a burden upon themselves as well as society.

Already, the demise is evident, that is in the gross loss of good, vital health. The pre-vaccination era pictures of Americans are highly revealing. All that is needed is to recall the robust, tall, dignified appearance of the early American pioneers. This is evident from any old photographs, which readily demonstrate the strength of these people. That was the pre-vaccination strength of the people. That strength has now been culled. No such vital health is seen today, perhaps except in unvaccinated immigrants. This is a crime beyond conception.

The degree of damage caused by vaccinations is beyond comprehension. The fact is vaccinations are a crime against humanity, perhaps the greatest of all crimes perpetrated by modern man. War kills, but so do vaccines, usually through a slow writhing death. In contrast, there is no evidence that vaccines cure disease. However, there is a plethora of evidence that they cause it, particularly neurological disorders and cancer.

It is difficult to dispel ingrained ideas. For Americans it is presumed that vaccines are necessary. It is also presumed that any opponent of this procedure is a radical, perhaps fanatic. Yet, do any of its proponents provide proof that vaccines are effective as well as safe? Perhaps it is the vaccine promoters who are the fanatics, since without documentation of safety they foist their wares upon the human race.

Can any such proponents refute their cancer-causing effects? Is there any evidence against the claim, fully documented by Japanese research, that in babies vaccines weaken the immune system or the American finding that pertussis, that is whooping cough, is more common in the vaccinated than those who refuse the vaccine? Or, can anyone dispute Dr. Hugh Fudenberg's analysis based upon data from the Mayo Clinic that repeated flu vaccines dramatically increase the risks for Alzheimer's disease or the finding of J. Anthony Morris, M.D. that merely inhaling the flu vaccine virus increases the growth rate of malignancies?

The evidence against the vaccine method is overwhelming. That it is an utter and absolute fraud seems difficult to dispute. In a civilized country where all the amenities of modern life are available and public hygiene is intact there is no sound basis for preventive immunization. Societies where sanitation and modern lifestyles are intact fail to need it. Without it there would be no major epidemics, plus the incidence of degenerative diseases, which are devastating Western nations, would plummet. The fact is the vaccination program is a financial ploy aimed perhaps at denuding the populations' health, all for perverse gains. Mass vaccinations have largely created an entire industry, that of cancer treatment, particularly in children, who are the primary victims of this procedure. Again, the fact that yearly in the United States and Canada alone thousands of children develop cancer directly as a result of vaccinations is undeniable.

But the government would never hurt us. . .

Regarding the claim that vaccines are safe there is no reason to believe it. This is largely because of the conflict of interest. In other words, the information is biased to suit a specific agenda. Financial interests are the only benchmark. The supreme authority on vaccinations, the CDC, is itself in conflict. According to a UPI article, July 2003, by Mark Benjamin: *UPI Investigates: The Vaccine Conflict*, the CDC cannot be regarded as an unbiased source. Said Benjamin:

> *Since the mid-1980s the (CDC) has doubled the number of vaccines children get, up to nearly 40 doses before age 2. The CDC also tracks possible side effects, along with the Food and Drug Administration. This puts the agency in the awkward position of evaluating the safety of its own recommendations. The CDC is in the vaccine business. Under a 1980 law, the CDC currently has 28 license agreements with companies and one university of vaccine or vaccine-related products. It has eight ongoing projects to collaborate on new vaccines...The situation...gives critics plenty of reason to worry that vaccine side effects are worse than CDC officials say.*

Jon Rappoport reports in his Web site, nomorefakenews.com, that the CDC, as well as the FDA, is well aware that vaccines are dangerous. This relates to the adverse reports system mandated by Congress for tracking any vaccine-induced reactions and/or deaths. Says Rappoport:

> *...the system contained 244,424 total reports of possible reactions to vaccines, including 98,145 emergency room visits, 5,149 life-threatening reactions, 27,925 hospitalizations, 5,775 disabilities, and 5,309 deaths...*

Incredibly, this data was compiled by the government's own researchers. Yet, these are only the reported cases. It is reasonable to presume that a equal number go unreported, in fact, a greater number. Parents may not realize that their child's sickness, a sudden temperature or cough, the sudden onset of behavioral disorders, an outbreak of skin rash or eczema, the catastrophic development of diabetes, could be vaccine-induced. Thus, reasonably this number is far higher than reported, perhaps, conservatively, ten times greater. This means that since the data was accumulated, about 1991 to date, there have been over two million reactions, with some 50,000 permanently disabled and some 40,000 deaths. Yet, this too is conservative. Rappoport reports that for adverse reactions filed by the FDA a realistic figure is to multiply the reported case 10-fold and even up to 100-fold.

Most people don't known that there is an adverse effects reporting system. Thus, in fact, since the early 1990s the total number of victims may never be known.

Yet, conservatively, since the reporting began a minimum of 25,000 people, many of whom were babies and children, have been killed by a therapy which is presumed as safe. In contrast, in the same period nutritional or herbal supplements have been associated with at a maximum thirty deaths, and this is over a period of nearly seventy years. 25,000 versus thirty: the individual can easily decide which direction to pursue. Even so, this fails to include the sudden deaths of children, that is SIDS, which are largely due to vaccinations. Here, it is a simple cause and effect: the child is healthy, receives the vaccine, and shortly thereafter (that is within a month or so), dies.

Yet, all this is preventable, since there is no need to treat children with dangerous medicines. Proper diet, healthy/natural nutritional supplements, plenty of natural vitamin C, and the appropriate herbal supplements, such as edible oil of wild Oreganol (P73) and Kid-e-Kare rubbing oil, will keep the baby/child healthy. Obviously, here breast-feeding is a mainstay. Should a person believe in the safety and effectiveness of highly contaminated injections or the safety and usefulness of a more natural approach, diet, nutrition, and high quality nutritional and herbal supplements? In contrast to the uncountable deaths yearly due to drugs and vaccines, there are essentially no childhood or infantile deaths known from food-grade herbal and nutritional supplements. The statistics tell all.

Thus, vaccines are a major cause of disability and death. Globally, every year thousands suddenly die from vaccine reactions. This means that in America the true number of deaths remains unknown. Only rarely are such deaths traced to vaccinations. Thousands more die from various chronic diseases, the result of the injection of foreign proteins, live germs, and germ genetic material.

Since vaccinations cause disease, including various types of cancer, is there any reason to continue prescribing them? It would seem that the use of any kind of vaccine is a fruitless endeavor, since, rather than preventing or curing diseases they cause them. Thus, they achieve the opposite of their purported claim-they are killers instead of cures.

Yet, the statistics for adverse effects fail to include another dire consequence: the toxicity of experimental vaccines. For instance, consider the vaccine for Lyme disease. This was tested initially on humans, without a scientific basis. The vaccine was approved by the CDC and within a year of its launch some 1.4 million individuals had been injected. However, due to adverse reactions which included dire inflammatory disorders, including Lyme disease-like syndromes and numerous deaths, it was rapidly pulled from the market.

How could such a dangerous vaccine be approved? Rappoport again discovers the answer:

> According to the CDC meeting transcripts where the advisory committee weighted its recommendation, five of the 10 committee members disclosed their financial conflicts of interest with vaccine manufacturers. Three of the five had conflicts of interest with SmithKlineBeecham (the manufacturer of the Lyme vaccine).

What a corrupt process it is: the people responsible for approving the vaccines were placed there by the drug companies. What's more, they knew they couldn't get approval. So, they stacked the committee. Thus, there is no possibility that such a vaccine was based upon accurate science. Rather, its release was based upon financial interests, yet, incredibly, dozens of people died from it. Regarding the hepatitis B vaccine the same disturbing conflict of interest is found. Says Rappoport:

> ...several of the health officials who took part, at the CDC in 1991, in recommending this vaccine for all newborn infants "had close ties to vaccine manufacturers." Dr. Sam Katz was chairman of this CDC committee in 1991. He also "worked as a paid consultant for Merck, Wyeth, and most major vaccine manufacturers." Merck manufactures a Hepatitis B vaccine. Another member of the CDC committee who endorsed the Hepatitis B vaccine for all babies was Dr. Neil Halsey. "Halsey...has done research paid for by most of the major vaccine manufacturers...he also established the John's Hopkins Institute of Vaccine Safety, started (with money) from several vaccine manufacturers..."

Yet, it is always represented that the medical profession is altruistic, that is the CDC is Americans' preventive medicine arm, modern medical doctors use "preventive vaccinations," etc. In contrast, it is assumed that the great medical men of the past were sleuths, true miracle men, whose only purpose was to save humankind. Far from it; rather, it would appear that their objective was/is fame and riches. Thus, in modern medicine there is no altruism.

Modern medicine has existed for about 100 years. Through it untold billions have been spent pursuing "cures." In all this searching not a single cure has been found. With the exception of perhaps the smallpox vaccine not a single synthetic drug or vaccine has proven curative for any disease. Yet, even with smallpox vaccines numerous early investigators claimed that the side effects were greater than any benefit. Many of such investigators recorded a greater number of deaths from the vaccine than the disease, that is the disease was cured but "the patient died."

Despite untold tens of billions spent there is no cure for the major killers, heart disease, high blood pressure, stroke, cancer, drug-resistant infections, and diabetes. Yet, the fantasy of the medical "miracle men" continues. It was L. E. Arnow, who demonstrated the degree of propaganda with the title of his book, *Health in a Bottle: Searching for Drugs that Help*. The subscript reads,"That we may live in better health and longer, we and our children use medicines, vaccines, injections." Yet, who was L. E. Arnow except the Director of Research for the pharmaceutical cartel, the holders of the patents for the drugs he touts.

Vaccine manufacturers have only one objective: to maintain global profits. Human health is never the issue. The government is also disinterested in human health, instead focusing on serving corporate interests. This dichotomy was apparently the concern of Senator Leahy, when he confronted President George W. Bush, Jr., about a provision in the so-called

Homeland Security Bill. In this bill a caveat was placed protecting an industry which has nothing to do with protecting lives. Rather, it protects only corporate interests, which perpetuate evil as well as cause premature death. The interaction between the Senator and the President is telling:

> MR. LEAHY. Mr. President, tucked away in the Homeland Security bill is a small provision that no one seems to want to take credit for and yet it would bestow benefits on just one interest group. According to news accounts, sections 714 through 716 of the Homeland Security bill were "Something the White House Wanted," not necessarily something the House or Senate wanted.

> This explanation hardly clarifies why we are including such a far-reaching amendment that has nothing to do with homeland security in this bill. It hardly explains why...we have decided to so blatantly put the interests of a few corporate pharmaceutical manufacturers before the interests of thousands of consumers, parents, and children.

> Sections 714, 715 and 716 basically give an "out of court free" card to Eli Lilly and other manufacturers of thimerasol...

> Parents and health professionals are now concerned that using vaccines with thimerasol has exposed 30 million American children to mercury levels far exceeding the "safe" level recommended by the Environmental Protection Agency. In 1999, the American Academy of Pediatrics and the Public Health Service began urging vaccine manufacturers to stop using thimerasol as quickly as possible. Since then, parents of autistic children have gone to court to hold

pharmaceutical companies liable for the alleged damage caused by thimerasol. Many of these parents now cite pharmaceutical manufacturers' own documents to show that they knew of the potential risk of using mercury-based preservatives back in the 1940s and yet did not stop its use.

Now, tucked away in the Homeland Security bill, we find this small provision that changes the definition of a vaccine manufacturer to include those companies that made vaccine preservatives. This small change to the Vaccine Injury Compensation program cuts the legs out from under the families involved in pending lawsuits against thimerasol manufacturers. The amendment is obvious in its attempt to put up roadblocks to these cases. Those who brought the cases against the manufacturers would lose their option of going to court while the manufacturers get new protections from large judgements.

Let's be clear about this provision. It has nothing to do with homeland security. We should not take the rights away of our citizenry under the guise of trying to protect them. (Interestingly, Senator Leahy was a recipient of an anthrax letter.)

This proves the entire Homeland Security Act is a fraud. Rather than for the people it is used against them. Thus, regarding this government mandate it is the general public which is its victim. What's more, the government has been using this act as a bludgeoning device against an entire people, that is the various Muslim populations. Have the Muslim populations, who are currently being attacked by the United States government, for instance, the people of Afghanistan, Palestine, and Iraq, ever caused harm to the

U.S. population? This is compelling proof of the evil nature of this plan. The fact is it is the 'Corporate-land' Security bill. Rather than protection against terrorism its purpose is to secure corporate profits regardless of the consequences, including the loss of the rights of citizens. Obviously, the profits of Eli Lilly have nothing to do with the security of the citizens. Nor do they have any connection with reducing terrorism. The fact is such a supposed protection is terrorism. By creating vast human harm, as well as harm to the environment, the manufacturers of thimerasol, including Eli Lilly and Aventis-Pasteur, have terrorized uncountable millions of beings, in fact, killing thousands of them. Plus, they have created another type of terror which is beyond measure: the epidemic of autism, mental retardation, and attention deficit. Thus, the true terrorists are the lawyers, who masquerade as politicians and create their own clique: their own set of laws for selfish interests.

Rather than some nebulous fringe element it is instead the greedy industrialists who are the proven terrorists. Thus, instead of protecting against it the Homeland Security Act foments terror. Entire diseases are due to mercury, including autism, attention deficit, mental retardation, psychosis, schizophrenia, neuropathy, Bell's palsy, epilepsy, dementia, and multiple sclerosis. Imagine the horror of living with such diseases—the pain and agony, the despair and death. This is terrorism. Yet, via the bill the true terrorist is protected: the very drug company which is largely responsible for numerous diseases. It calls into question the entire bill as having little if anything to do with protecting U.S. citizens, rather, clearly, as sited by Senator Leahy the citizens are the victims, in fact, they are being terrorized by it. This proves that the bill is a corruption of the most vast degree. The public gains no benefit from it: only harm. The fact is the so-called War on Terror is merely a ruse for disguising the true criminals—the hierarchy of the American and Israeli governments.

The question is who on the Board of Eli Lilly and its associates is, simultaneously, vested in the White House? This will tell the real source of this bill, which calls for continued harm to the American public, not its protection. Thus, the Homeland Security Act is a fraud, created long before the 9/11 debacle for the benefit of the vested few. Criminals, the creators of this provision seem oblivious to the unmerciful harm they create, as is demonstrated by the following report of a thimerasol victim:

> Keaan East...was a happy, healthy two-year old, who "achieved every developmental milestone expected of all normally developing children," says a lawsuit filed against vaccine maker Aventis-Pasteur. But something went wrong, alleges the suit, after Keaan received at least three shots of the DPT vaccine. "He stopped talking and only made sounds," the suit says. "He became unresponsive and withdrawn and made no eye contact. He started injuring himself by banging his head against objects and biting his hands." the suit...blames Thimerasol, an ethyl-mercury derivative used to preserve vaccines. The suit says mercury is particularly toxic to infants and the parents were never told it was used in the vaccines. Yet another victim is Amanda McCullough, who suffered a sudden shock reaction after a DPT vaccine. According to her mother, Anna McCullough, Amanda was a "happy, healthy baby" who turned "grey and lifeless" within an hour after the vaccination. She was rushed to the hospital and resuscitated, but she began having uncontrolled seizures. Amanda survived but continues to have seizures, which require large amounts of medication.

Yet, the Homeland, that is Corporateland, Security Act primarily indemnifies Eli Lilly from any public redress. Again, how does this ensure the peoples' security? The fact is it diminishes public safety. Lilly is well aware that its highly dangerous DPT vaccine caused uncountable disability, retardation, disease, and death. This is the same company which makes Vioxx, also responsible for much death and devastation.

Regardless of the consequences the government chooses to preferentially place its shroud around this corporation, this maker of killer drugs. Yet, it is the government, that is those vested individuals with financial ties, who are themselves liable. Such individuals use their position in public trust to protect, in fact, advance, their personal finances. In other words, by protecting Vioxx they are/were protecting their own selves: all at the peoples' expense. This is a crime of the greatest degree. The fact is this is precisely the motivation for the aforementioned provisions. Because of Thimersol Lilly is under the siege of lawsuits from all over the world.

The government has attempted to neutralize these suits or, at least, so the claimants are led to believe. What the government has done is illegal. It is terrorism against the masses. This is because rather than the public it is elected to serve, the purpose of the provision was only to protect personal and/or financial interests.

There is a telling connection: a top government official in the Bush administration is an Eli Lilly V. P.: Mitch Daniels, Director of the Office of Management and Budget. There is an even more revelatory connection: Senator Bill Frist. Even before the Homeland Security Act was 'enacted' this former surgeon attempted to pass a bill protecting Lilly from lawsuits for its crimes. He also foisted upon Americans legislation for additional vaccines, which, in fact, was thwarted by Senator Kennedy. The fact is Frist is a medical doctor. It is in his interest to pursue the vaccine agenda. Frist is indelibly tied to the very agenda he promotes.

According to William Rivers Pitt, *New York Times* columnist and noted author, Frist's only reasons to support this position are due to financial interests. The fact is he is in politics to maintain his family fortune. His family, says Pitt, is vested in the pharmaceutical business, whose fortune was made in the massive and corrupt HMO, Hospital Corporation of America. Lilly is a great contributor to this corporation. Incredibly, this is the individual who makes the laws regarding what is best for Americans.

Many of the people who work there own stock in Lilly. Frist, who receives financial aid from this company, denies any knowledge of the thimerasol provision. The White House also denies any knowledge. Yet, it was constructed within the White House specifically for Lilly's benefit. Yet, it was George Walker Bush, father of former President George Bush, Sr., who during the 1970s was a long-standing member of Lilly's board. Surely, then, the Bush family would feel obligated to urge protection. This family has no interest of any sort in protecting American citizens.

Regarding the writing in of the Lilly clause, surely, this was a White House decision. The fact is the Bushs, Jr. and Sr., have directly benefitted from their associations with this company. Bush Sr. persistently lobbied on Lilly's behalf to the government for tax breaks. What's more, the Bush family is a major Lilly stockholder. Pitt also reports that disgraced Enron CEO Kenneth Lay was also a Board member. There is an even more direct connection. During the 2002 election period, says Pitt, "Eli Lilly gave more campaign money—1.6 million—than any other pharmaceutical corporation, 79% of which went to Republican candidates." Thus, at a minimum the Lilly amendment is a political favor for campaign funds. In other words, Lilly purchased the right for high crimes. However, there is another objective: the protection of personal fortunes. This is terrorism to the highest degree. In other words, through its political connections Lilly purchased the right to continue poisoning Americans, in fact, people globally. Thus, it becomes clear that the War on Terror is a fraud, because its purpose is never to protect the masses. Rather, it is to further specific corporate agendas, including the interests of war contractors.

Because of Lilly's oppressive procedures people die. Yet, the supposedly protective Homeland Security Act attempts to ensure that this company continues to wreak havoc upon the populace, particularly regarding thimerasol poisoning of infants and children. This is without restriction—without even an iota of accountability—to murder people, and this is deemed security? All this is for profits. There is no caring for the people. Rather than security this is tyranny.

Chapter 10
Foreign Invaders

It has been long known that the injection of foreign matter into the body is dangerous. A mere splinter creates an obvious reaction. The immune system essentially attacks it, creating inflammation, redness, and swelling. There is great pain and the possibility for spread of infection, even a dangerous infection, that is unless the splinter is removed. Incredibly, the same process occurs when any foreign substance is injected in the body, and this includes the ingredients in vaccines.

Vaccines were formerly known as serums. This is a more accurate term than vaccines. This is because vaccines truly are a kind of animal blood, that is protein, matter. Thus, the term serum is synonymous with vaccine. An early book written C. F. von Pirquet, M. D., a German specialist, describes the dire concerns of physicians regarding vaccinations. Called *Serum Sickness* it describes in detail the vast biochemical and physiological derangement resulting from such injections. Then, in the early to mid-1900s serums, that is vaccines, were well known to cause systemic, that is dangerous, reactions. Extensive research was done to determine the consequences of the injection of foreign protein, that is the protein from the blood of various animals.

Vaccines are a kind of bloody material, so the reactions heretofore described may be deemed synonymous.

The whole idea of injecting materials of animal origin, particularly animal blood or serum, was originated by Europeans. As early as 1691 a German, Jungker, attempted to treat various diseases through the injection of lamb's blood. This practice continued for nearly a century, although it was found to largely be useless. Then, in Europe in the beginning of the 19th century it was again attempted, this time with catastrophic results. The "intravenous injections of lamb blood were soon found to be very dangerous." There was high fever, bleeding, blood clots, strokes, and sepsis. There was liver and kidney failure. Then, it was discovered that such injections caused a massive immune response, leading to a wide range of destructive processes. Thus, it was concluded there was no benefit in such a treatment. After numerous catastrophes, including multiple human deaths, the injection of animal fluids was "given up."

In 1894 the situation changed with the introduction of a serum-based treatment for diphtheria. This was prepared by the injection of horses with diphtheria "toxin" and, therefore, protein. Then, the horse lymph, which was, obviously, infected with germs, was harvested and injected into humans. The reactions with this serum were less severe, largely because this was a true serum, containing a low content of cells, like white and red blood cells. When blood was injected directly, the massive reactions seen then were largely the consequence of the vast amount of protein injected. Even so, despite its more liquefied nature serum sickness did occur, and, as a result, various illnesses developed, that is due to the injections. In contrast, it appeared that the injection offered benefit, and, so, serums regained popularity. However, that toxic reactions occurred, as well as chronic disease, is well documented.

Incredibly, people were under the impression that the antitoxin was a 'clean' serum, merely containing the needed antidote. They failed to realize that the injection was a true serum derived from the blood of horses. Thus, it contained an unknown array of proteins as well as germs. German researchers eventually proved that the toxic reactions were due to massive systemic reactions to the various animal-source proteins found in horse blood. Such blood is foreign to the body. Obviously, the injection of such a substance will cause severe reactions. Typical symptoms of horse serum intoxication included rashes, joint pain, fever, eczema-like lesions, hives, and joint swelling as well as shock and sudden death.

These symptoms are obviously due to toxicity. This toxicity occurs in the form of a harsh immune reaction against the proteins. This is because the immune system regards them as poisons. It was Hamburger and Moro who in their landmark study showed that the injection of any kind of foreign protein into the bloodstream is abnormal. Interestingly, this is the very method used by allergists to determine reactions, the so-called scratch test. So, it is expected that if foreign protein—and this is precisely what vaccines are—is injected, there will be a toxic reaction.

This cannot be good for health. This was the investigator's conclusion, when in review of Hamburger and Moro's work, he said, "human beings produce precipitins after an injection of foreign serum." In other words, the human immune system attempts to purge these proteins from the blood. There is obviously a "great difference between parenteral (That is intravenous or intramuscular) and enteral (that is through the gut) introduction of foreign protein...the foreign protein is assimilated if taken by the normal physiological (that is through the intestinal) route, whereas if introduced in the...genetically abnormal way...it produced antibodies and *reactions in the form of disease.*"

Vaccine manufacturers fail to provide information on the possible reactions to vaccines. Nor do they explain the physiology. Yet, as early as the late 1800s these processes were well documented by German and Austrian physicians. What's more, such physicians regarded these reactions as disease processes, not the flippantly proclaimed "mild or insignificant reactions" attested to by the pharmaceutical houses. According to von Pirquet the injection of animal fluids, as found in vaccines, leads to a localized swelling, but this swelling may extend into the lymph glands, causing soreness, swelling, inflammation, redness, and pain. The injection site may become red with reddish blisters or pimples and often itches. Hives may develop, and they may be partly pale, that is they are not always beet red and itchy. In some people there may be no such reactions; there may only be a slight swelling of the lymph nodes. Usually, such reactions occur about 7 to 8 days and up to two weeks after the injection.

A temperature may develop. There may also be an outbreak of a systemic rash, which may or may not be itchy. Kidney damage is significant and is largely due to the toxic interaction of the foreign protein with protective immune proteins. These proteins collide to form antibody-antigen complexes, described as precipitins in earlier research, and as the name implies these complexes precipitate in the blood. The result is a clogging of kidney function, which causes edema.

Of note the authors call this reaction a disease. Thus, they demonstrate that vaccines are disease-producing. The swelling may be observed throughout the body, especially in the legs and under the eyes. Within days the swelling usually disappears. Rarely, there can be albumin in the urine, which is a sign of mild kidney damage. Joint pain is also common, and this may be permanent. There may also be residual kidney damage. Incredibly, the toxicity is so high that from a single vaccine an individual may gain one to two pounds of fluid weight.

In blood chemistry there is a bizarre finding, which defies the very purpose of these injections: a systematic decline in white blood cell count. In some cases a single vaccination can cause the white cell count to plummet to dangerously low levels. Von Piquet describes this as a highly abnormal, even toxic, reaction.

Von Pirquet emphasizes that there is an incubation period regarding such vaccinations. The reaction may not occur immediately. Usually, it begins about seven days after the injection, although in some cases the reaction may occur virtually immediately.

There may also be delayed reactions, occurring two weeks to two months post-injection. The greater the number of injections taken, as, for instance, the multiple injections given simultaneously to babies and children, the sooner and greater will be the reaction.

There is great danger in simultaneous multiple injections. He proves this, stating that while a single injection may prove tolerable multiple or repeated ones can cause significant disease. What's more, children or babies who receive repeated injections will likely show sudden or overnight reactions compared to those who receive single injections. Thus, regarding highly toxic reactions to pediatric vaccines, such as the DPT and MMR, it may not be immediate or even within a few days. There is an incubation period before the crisis strikes. That could be up to one month or more post-vaccination.

Von Pirquet demonstrates a monumental finding, largely neglected by today's physicians. This relates to a drop in body temperature. Vaccines derived from animal matter are highly destructive to the immune system. This is to such a degree that they damage body temperature regulation, causing a significant drop in normal temperature. Thus, it is no surprise that a low body temperature and lack of fever during illness are frequent symptoms of chronic viral infection.

The fact that vaccines cause a drop in body temperature is an ominous sign, that is of extreme dysregulation. It is a sign that the vaccine or serum has caused a depression of the immune and hormone systems. In innumerable cases the same pattern developed. After vaccination the normal body temperature is disrupted, and thereafter the person suffers a chronically low body temperature. This is highly dangerous, since it is the body temperature which helps strengthen immune function and assists in the purging of germs.

A normal body temperature aids in the production of critical immune components such as the white blood cells, lymphocytes, lymphatic secretions, platelets, interferon, and immunoglobulins. A high body temperature in response to an illness dramatically aids in the synthesis of white blood cells and other critical immune components. A low temperature causes a decline in such synthesis. Thus, a chronically low body temperature, which is the consequence of multiple vaccines, leads to a state of chronic immune suppression. This leaves the body highly vulnerable to the development of infectious diseases as well as cancer.

The digestive system can also be harshly affected by vaccinations. Von Pirquet documented numerous digestive symptoms, particularly relating to the colon. Mucousy and malformed stools, as well as diarrhea, were common. This is another sign of the highly toxic nature of these procedures. The fact is the epidemic in the West of colonic disorders, such as colitis, irritable bowel, Crohn's disease, and ulcerative colitis, may be largely related to vaccinations. There may also be a loss of appetite; the child is converted from a robust eater to a picky irritable eater. Obviously, as a result of serums and vaccines there is failure to thrive. In fact, in modern society vaccination is perhaps the primary cause of this syndrome. A child who suddenly does poorly in growth, stature, appetite, spinal development, and mental function is likely vaccine-intoxicated.

It is important to note that in some cases the swelling of the lymph glands can be extreme. Usually, the swelling in these nodes recedes. However, occasionally, they remain chronically swollen, and unless the lymphatic system is purged cancer may result. Due to the toxicity of the vaccination components the lymphatics may also become fibrotic.

The lymph glands fiercely attempt to process the invaders. However, if they are overwhelmed and the irritant or infectious agent persists, gross disease may result. Thus, contrary to the proclamations of the vaccine industry swollen lymph glands are unhealthy. The swellings must be eradicated through the proper natural medical care, for instance, the topical and internal use of spice oils, particularly oil of wild oregano (P73), and Kid-e-Kare rubbing oil. This is because such oils are potent lymphatic cleansers.

An oil of cold-pressed garlic could also prove invaluable for mobilizing and cleansing lymphatic fluids. Known as Garlex this cold-pressed mountain-grown garlic oil is the ideal formula for activating the lymphatics. Rich in naturally occurring sulfur it nourishes the tissues, while cleansing toxins and purging germs. It is the ideal adjunct to wild oregano therapy. This is to be taken internally. Enzymes also open up the lymphatic channels, that is ZymaClenz.

The lymph glands swell because of the direct toxicity of noxious proteins, harsh chemicals, and dangerous germs. Such toxins must be purged from the body, so that the lymphatic system can be normalized.

The internal organs may also be adversely affected, particularly those with lymphatic functions such as the spleen and liver. These organs may noticeably swell. Cell death may occur as well as inflammation. The thymus is adversely affected and, usually, it shrinks in size. Here too, cell death occurs. Great strain is also endured by the bone marrow, where cells undergo dramatic and potentially dangerous genetic changes. There is a gross increase in cell synthetic activity and reproduction but in an uncontrolled fashion. Is this to any degree synonymous with a cure?

Today, toxic reactions to vaccines are rarely realized. Doctors fail to measure this toxicity, largely because they vaccinate at such a young age. In such youngsters it is difficult to measure this toxicity through the blood. They also fail to recognize the development of vaccine-related illnesses, including eczema, psoriasis, and asthma. Yet, for any teenager or adult who must undergo vaccination measuring the pre- and post- white counts, hopefully as often as feasible, is essential. Von Pirquet showed that vaccines cause extreme toxicity to these cells. A decline of as much as 70% may occur. Such a decline is always a sign of disease, that is of fulminant toxicity. There can be no benefit to a medicine which causes such wholesale damage.

His conclusion is that as a result of the injection of animal-source fluids, rich in protein, massive systemic reactions occur. These reactions lead to cell damage, noticeably in the bone marrow, lymph glands, white blood cells, liver, and kidneys. The body falls into a depressed mode, while the white blood cell count, as well as the body temperature, drops. In reviewing his work it becomes evident that the body is unable to cope with such an insult and that this insult is always destructive.

Contrary to drug company literature there is no evidence that the injection of foreign protein from, for instance, a monkey, dog, mouse, human, horse, cow, or calf is safe. Nor is there any evidence that the repeated injection of vaccines or the injection of multiple vaccines, for instance, the DPT or MMR, is advantageous. Rather, such procedures, as he demonstrates, increase the immune system's aggression, accelerating the risks for dangerous reactions.

With vaccines there is an additive effect. This is why the majority of extreme reactions and/or fatalities occur after multiple injections. Thus, with each vaccine the potential for a sudden reaction dramatically increases. The body simply fails to be able to handle repeated toxic loads. What's more, this is precisely what an immunization is: a poisonous injection, which alters the way the immune system functions. This alteration is rarely if ever for the individual's benefit. Rather, it disrupts the biological systems, which increases the vulnerability to chronic disease.

Only one conclusion can be made from von Pirquet's work. Vaccines fail to support the immune system in any observable way. Rather, the research shows that they suppress it and even cause mass immune cell death. A single vaccine is capable of destroying billions of white blood cells. Multiple vaccines can completely disrupt white blood cell synthesis, while poisoning the bone marrow. In susceptible individuals this can lead to immune deficiency, inflammatory disorders, lymphoma, and leukemia. It was Mendelsohn who repeatedly observed that leukemia, now a Western epidemic, is the result of childhood vaccines. Of note prior to mass vaccinations no such epidemic existed.

The injection of animal proteins in babies creates great strain on their bodies. Their delicate and poorly formed immune systems are incapable of reversing this stress—the fact is even adults are incapable of withstanding it. That the infant immune system is inadequate is fully demonstrated by the proven side effects as well as fulminant diseases such as inflammation of the brain, respiratory disorders, and severe allergic reactions. For those who remain skeptical about such side effects realize that the majority of these adverse effects are published by the vaccine makers themselves. These may be found in medical textbooks, drug company inserts, and the PDR.

Whenever serums or foreign proteins are injected into the body, the immune system attacks them. This leads to the formation of clumps of protein known as antigen-antibody complexes. The antigens are the foreign proteins; the antibodies are the secretions of the immune system, which neutralize them. The formation of antigen-antibody complexes helps prevent further toxicity of the invaders and in the case of germs, attack on the internal organs. In infants and newborns in particular the ability to form antigen-antibody complexes is diminished. Thus, when foreign substances are injected, particularly germs, damage to the internal organs, as well as systemic infection, are likely. Due to the immature condition there is no firm immune defense against this. This makes immunizations far more dangerous in newborns and infants than any other age group. There may not be death but there is certainly chronic inflammation and infection, which may lead to a variety of conditions which, normally, would not be associated with injections.

Consider the hepatitis B vaccine, which is given at birth. This vaccine has been associated with an enormous range of disorders, which are largely due to organ damage and inflammation. Parents would never realize the connections. Such hepatitis B vaccine-induced diseases include diabetes, thyroid dysfunction, Addison's disease, brain inflammation (resulting in retardation, seizures, etc.), meningitis, chronic bronchitis, asthma, multiple sclerosis-like illnesses, memory loss, arthritis, autoimmune disorders (including Hashimoto's thyroiditis, liver disorders, disorders of the spleen, epilepsy, and paralysis. In particular, it is a major cause of sudden-onset diabetes. This is proof that the components of the injection remain at large, fully escaping any immune defense. Then, this toxicity progresses, leading to acute or chronic disease.

Then, is the individual to believe the claim that this vaccine, injected into defenseless American babies, is safe? Medical authorities claim that reactions to the vaccine are rare. In contrast, as reported by Tim O'Shea it was Jane Orient, M.D., Director of the Association of American Physicians, who called for an immediate withdrawal of the vaccine. Said Orient deaths and toxic reactions to the vaccine are "vastly underreported, as formal long-term studies of vaccine safety have not been completed."

The challenge for parents is that due to the immature nature of the newborn/infant's immune system after a vaccine reaction may not occur immediately, that is an obvious one. It may take days, weeks, or even months—even years—for the full scope of the toxicity to be revealed. Generally, the greater the number of vaccinations the sooner will be the physiological collapse. What's more, if these injections are given in close proximity, then the reaction may be sudden. Studies reported by von Pirquet show that on average a reaction cannot be expected for some 5 to 6 days, with the majority occurring 8 to 14 days after the injection. Again, for repeated injections or injections given simultaneously, such as the multiple-dose childhood vaccines, the likelihood for a reaction is greatly increased. Here, it essentially occurs immediately. Yet, if the immune system is naturally strong, there may be no noticeable reaction or the reaction is such that the newborn or infant seemingly recovers. Yet, the infecting agent(s) has been delivered and remains unscathed. Then, eventually, there develops chronic disease. However, usually, no one associates it with vaccinations.

This coincides with the statistics reported by O'Shea, that is that severe toxic reactions, in fact, deaths, occurred in infants primarily within one to four weeks after vaccination, in this instance, with the DPT. The mechanism was again confirmed by von Pirquet, who found that after injecting serums (that is vaccines), the amount of toxins, which he called precipitins, in the blood could be measured. For instance, following a single injection he found the toxins to be "abundant" about eleven days post-vaccination, while for repeated vaccinations at the fifth day levels were high.

The materials he measured, the highly toxic antigen-antibody complexes, are capable of causing widespread damage, including blood clots, stroke, allergic shock, and kidney damage. This merely demonstrates that as a result of repeated vaccinations sudden reactions are much more common, and, thus, the risk for fatality is far greater as a result of multiple vaccinations.

That immunization is the cause of the symptoms, notes von Pirquet, is beyond doubt. Were it not for the vaccine there would be no such reactions. Doctors claim vaccinations as a medical breakthrough, because they improve the immune defenses. Thus, they have hailed the injection of foreign proteins as a necessary evil. They have proclaimed this method "safe and effective." It is precisely the boost the immune system requires, they attest, so that humankind is protected from the ravages of disease. Von Pirquet disputes this. As a result of careful scientific studies he proclaims that the foreign proteins, rather than benefitting the immune system, poison it, that is:

...the antigen (that is the foreign protein injected through vaccinations)...elicits symptoms (of the disease).

Thus, von Pirquet demonstrates the opposite, that disease is the consequence of vaccines. This is what careful, cautious research proves. The vaccine makers have no such research. The fact is they are unable to prove that their wares are safe.

Von Pirquet demonstrates another critical finding, which largely explains the destructive nature of vaccines. He determined that in humans the opposite of what was expected occurred. Often, people who were the sickest were those who had little if any measurable antigen-antibody complexes, while those who had high levels of such complexes tended to recover more readily. In one case he describes a vaccinated individual who had the "most intensive symptoms...showing only traces (of these complexes)..." This demonstrates the diabolical nature of vaccines. Obviously, in this case the test subject's prolonged illness was due to a stealth infection, which escaped immune reaction. This is the origin of chronic disease, which may afflict the recipient for life.

Yet, perhaps his most compelling finding is the nature of the very basis of the foreign protein/germ and immune system reactions. This relates to the claim by vaccine makers that vaccinations modulate the immune response, that is they 'work' with immunity to eliminate the risk for infection—that they cause the immune system to develop a specialized immunity against the injected germ. This concept is used to justify any reactions as a "normal immune response" and that "reactions are a good sign of a strong immune reaction." Von Pirquet provides evidence against this. He found that the injection of animal proteins, as found in common vaccines, fails to elicit natural immunity. Rather than an immune response the proteins themselves were toxic, and the common reactions, such as swelling at the injection site, edema, pain inflammation, fever, chills, muscle, and joint pain, are due to the poison itself. In other words, other than any immune boosting, all the symptoms from vaccines are due to the injection of these animal-source drugs. Obviously, vaccines poison the cells.

This would indicate that the entire basis of immunization is fraudulent. According to von Pirquet in some 35% of test subjects the immune system did virtually nothing: the full spectrum of the symptoms were due to the injected toxins, that is the direct toxic action of the injected proteins. Thus, the toxicity and, therefore, symptoms, occurred independent of any immune response. This is an incredible finding, which fully disables the argument of a positive consequence from the injections. Von Pirquet makes it clear that, in fact, serums are toxic and that as a result of their injection entire diseases may develop. In contrast to today's medical authorities, he regards the entire process resulting from vaccinations, whether there is a potent immune response or not, as poisonous.

Many serums and vaccines are commercially weakened, to minimize a sudden, noticeable immune reactions. Such vaccines are called "attenuated", which, in fact, means weakened. Tests by von Pirquet demonstrated that even these weakened or diluted serums are toxic. He said,

> In a diluted solution reactions are slowed down. The formation of the toxic substances does not take place with one stroke but is distributed over a longer period of time. Thus its effect does not reach the threshold of clinical detectibility.

In other words, no obvious reaction can be seen, and, thus, it is virtually impossible to trace the source of the negative effects. These effects may become manifested months, years, or decades after the injection(s).

That vaccines cause brain damage is beyond dispute. Tests on rabbits are revealing. Through injecting animal proteins, as well as germ residues, into the animals the danger became obvious:

> A rabbit (was) pretreated with 8 injections... Approximately one minute later the animal made movements like sneezing, became anxious and restless, lay down on its abdomen; breathing became rapid...Many bowel movements set in, then the rabbit lay on its side turned the head back, made running movements with the paws and finally remained motionless, (until)...respiration stopped.

These are toxic reactions from the serum of mere herbivores: horses. Yet, it would appear that there developed a type of 'mad rabbit' disease. What's more, what could be expected from the derivatives of a carnivorous or more aggressive types of animal such as monkeys? Monkeys are primarily herbivores, but, like pigs, they may also eat meat, even each other. Thus, their blood chemistry will be different than that of a horse and/or cow, in fact, far more disease-ridden. What's more, monkeys are tropical animals, and, certainly, are not an edible species. Thus, it would be expected that, genetically, the human immune system would be unfamiliar with monkey proteins and that it would, therefore, react violently to this invasion. Or, at a minimum, surely, bizarre and unnatural proteins would cause tissue damage even chronic disease.

Monkey serum: fraud upon humanity

That tens of millions of Americans would be injected or caused to swallow components of monkey tissue as well as blood, is incomprehensible. This was supposedly under the guise of scientific research. In their push for the vaccine the perpetrators served exclusively their own agendas. Evidence of public concern is nonexistent. For instance, Salk used the money and notoriety he received to create his own research and financial empire. The March of Dimes foundation became a national icon. These are the beneficiaries, while the public suffered grotesquely. The fact is it is not possible to indiscriminately inject a population with a group of bizarre foreign proteins and pathogens from such a disease-ridden animal, caged wild rhesus monkeys, without causing catastrophes. This is precisely what occurred. It is a catastrophe which continues to haunt tens of millions of people.

There are those who would be skeptical of these claims. Yet, any reasonable individual would at least question the safety of injecting components of monkey blood, even monkey sperm, saliva, and urine, into the human body. An early monograph, "Care and Diseases of the Research Monkey," published in the *Annals of the New York Academy of Sciences*, 1960, is revealing. This is the era of the polio virus research on these creatures. The first chapter deals with the transportation of monkeys, citing the many problems. Incredibly, this chapter is authored by the notorious Eli Lilly through one of its executives, Donald DeValois.

Initially, it is noted, the transportation is wrought with catastrophes, largely due to the bizarre and frightening change of the monkey's environment from total freedom to a caged existence. This obviously creates vast problems, primarily of nutrition and sanitation. In the wild monkeys notoriously maintain great space between each other, jealously guarding their territories. Thus, placing monkeys in closed spaces dramatically impugns their health. Routinely, captive monkeys defecate and urinate on themselves, while also defecating and urinating on their food. Then, they eat that food.

First, the monkey must be trapped in the wild. Then, there is usually a transfer to a bamboo crate. Says DeValois:

> This cage is never cleaned or sanitized, and is replaced with a new one only when it is no longer serviceable. Thus, the newly trapped monkey encounters his first experience with excretions and secretions of monkeys outside his own family group...the newly captured monkeys are placed in larger bamboo slat crates measuring 36 by 60 by 30 inches high. Twenty animals are normally kept in this crate. Water is supplied in a large crock, and feed grain is sprinkled on the ground...Contamination of the grain with waste materials is obvious, and each animal directly contacts secretions and excretions from a few more animal contacts. Both these factors are significant heath problems, along with the fact that the diet frequently is inadequate...

Then, what happens next is incredible. The animals are sold in the open market and then shipped by train to a monkey farm, where they are sorted and held. There (in what is now known as New Delhi, India,) up to 300 monkeys were put together in a room-sized pen. For any wild beast this is a highly abnormal and stressful circumstance. The pen is "sanitized once each week." Lilly's DeValois continues:

> Animals generally remain at the farm from 2 to 10 days while a planeload of 1800 animals is being assembled. When the monkeys have been examined and selected for shipment to the United States they are packed into a wooden shipping crate measuring 21 by 36 by 19 inches. Seven large or nine small monkeys are placed in each crate. The loaded crates are transported to the Delhi airport...
>
> Once aboard the aircraft en route to the United States, monkeys seem to travel well if they are comfortable. The metabolism and waste products of 1800 monkeys put a considerable strain on an airplane ventilation system designed to keep 80 to 100 human passengers comfortable. Further complications arise from the fact that the plane travels through and tops at climactic areas ranging from the tropical to arctic. Consequently, potential problems of temperature, humidity, and air movement are continuously presented...(in certain climates)...a great deal of cold air can at times pour in on the animals in the crates...

Obviously, under such conditions the animals develop illnesses, which rapidly spread in the "monkey colony." DeValois continues, claiming that the cages became contaminated with feces and urine throughout the flight, and so did the drinking water. Finally, the monkeys arrived in Indianapolis, where Eli Lilly is housed, and were transported to its facility. By this time their health is extensively compromised, and disease sets in.

Once under the drug company's auspices the fate of the monkeys is dire. Already stressed from the inhumane changes, they are highly agitated and frightened. This makes them toxic. They are sick, infected by their own wastes and the wastes of other monkeys. They develop a variety of infections, including abscesses (that is pus-pockets). Then, they are descended upon by a team of doctors, and, thus, they endure further pain. With potent drugs they are tranquilized, and minor surgeries are performed. As a routine drugs are added to their feed, and by injection they are sedated. A wide range of antibiotics and antiparasitic agents are given. Secondary fungal infections due to the antibiotics are common.

Monkey virus B: the monkey bite agent

The manipulation of monkeys or monkey tissues has long been known as a dangerous endeavor. A particularly aggressive monkey virus was first isolated from the nerve tissue of a deceased lab worker, who died after being bitten by a lab monkey. The existence of this virus, different from the SV40, then known as monkey B virus, alone should have put the fear of God in the researchers. This sufficiently should have prevented further research.

Since the danger of monkey viruses was well published at a minimum there should have been a moratorium on any direct exposure of humans to monkey-derived materials. Since the dangers of human exposure to monkey tissues were so well known, how did an industry flourish while relying upon monkey organs for making drugs? It was well known that even the slightest contact with a caged monkey, a mere scratch, let alone a bite, could result in death. In the 1950s

Keeble reported that in the rhesus monkeys which were used to make the polio vaccine, "the disease is widespread." Some researchers found that all monkeys are infected with a polio-like virus, only a more aggressive form.

The virulence is increased by antibiotic therapy, which all captive monkeys are subjected to. Monkey virus B is not only a highly aggressive germ, it is readily communicable. The mere injection or oral intake of the virus, as, for instance, in a vaccine derived from rhesus monkeys, causes infection. In such a scenario the virus will likely cause chronic disease, particularly neurological disorders such as ALS, multiple sclerosis, Parkinson's disease, dementia, and Alzheimer's disease. Early manifestations of the infection include ulcerations on the tongue, cold sores, canker sores, trigeminal neuralgia, tics, and Bell's palsy. This is due to the infection of the nerves by the virus, which resides in the brain, brain stem, and spinal cord. The fact is this germ is highly aggressive in its ability to attack nerve tissues, including the brain and spinal nerves. It is likely a major cause of demyelination diseases, that is diseases where the nerve sheaths are attacked and destroyed. Is it possible that the epidemic of such diseases, particularly multiple sclerosis, is a monkey virus consequence?

Acute infection due to direct inoculation of the virus through contact with laboratory animals is rare. Usually, as a result of such contact death results. The majority of these deaths are due to massive infection of the brain. That the polio vaccines were contaminated with this virus, though in an altered form, is indisputable. This is exemplified by the case of a laboratory worker, who in 1958 while working on the polio vaccine was infected. His accident record "revealed that on two occasions he had suffered minor lacerations of his hands from broken glass containing tissue cultures of monkey renal (that is kidney) cells."

First, he developed symptoms of an upper respiratory infection...he complained of a persistent cough for approximately five weeks. Then, after improving temporarily he developed chills and stiffness of the neck. Complications rapidly developed, his temperature rose dramatically and, then, he improved. Yet, suddenly, he became cyanotic and died. The pathology report revealed systematic infection of the brain, that is viral encephalitis. Monkey virus B was isolated from brain tissue and identified. This was the original reported case of infection not from direct contact with live monkeys but, rather, from the tissue cultures used for human research. Thus, clearly, the pharmaceutical cultures used to make human vaccines were/are infected. The number of children who were likely infected by this virus cannot be counted, but it surely amounts to millions, perhaps hundreds of millions.

The virus remains in remission in the brain and spinal cord, only to surface as a result of a toxic insult: severe prolonged stress, drug therapy, cortisone, a spinal tap, surgery, general anesthesia, or similar traumas. Then, when it arises, it can cause unmerciful degenerative diseases.

There were many other cases due to direct contact with monkeys or monkey bites/scrapes. In many of these cases the symptoms resemble common human conditions, particularly multiple sclerosis and sudden paralysis. Could these disorders be due to monkey virus B? Could chronic neurological disorders, which develop post-vaccination, such as autism, attention deficit, mental retardation, epilepsy, and schizophrenia, also be due to this virus? Could this virus also induce cancer? This is highly likely. This virus resides in monkey blood and any blood derivative such as the polio vaccines and even some modern vaccines originating from rhesus monkeys.

Virtually anyone who received a polio vaccine has the infection. In other words, all vaccine batches were likely infected. The virus survivedsterilization techniques. SV40 fully resists treatment with both mercurial compounds and formaldehyde. Apparently, the B virus, which is, essentially, the monkey form of the human herpes virus, is equally resistant to chemical treatment. Surely, this virus too survived the formaldehyde/mercury treatment and is living today in uncountable humans. If it is alive, it must be infecting them. The fact is this is a demyelinating virus, which creates a disease picture similar to multiple sclerosis. It also creates an encephalitis-like disease. Thus, in certain demyelinating diseases in which herpetic viruses are implicated, including ALS, multiple sclerosis, myasthenia gravis, Parkinson's disease, autoimmune disorders, and Alzheimer's disease, monkey viruses may be implicated, surely SV40 and perhaps the herpetic cousin, monkey virus B.

In such diseases the brain is under attack. There is destruction of its outer coating. The nerves of the spinal cord are also destructively attacked. Viruses flourish in nerve tissue, and this is certainly true of monkey viruses. All such diseases were rare in the pre-vaccination era, many of which were essentially unknown. The fact is through the administration of non-tested or experimental vaccines human beings have been infected with organisms unknown; only a few of the possible pathogens have been identified.

Regarding vaccines there is no proof they are germ-free. The fact is they are derived from germ-infested materials which harbor countless species of microbes. Animal blood and other secretions are notoriously contaminated with germs. SV40 and monkey virus B are among the few which have been discovered. These germs now live within humans, who pass them through the generations. The fact is these germs are carcinogens which perpetuate the cancer epidemic. Thus, in order to protect the self, as well as the future generations, they must be purged. This is achieved through the regular intake of the potent germicide, P73, both as the oil and aromatic essence. The power of this purge is demonstrated by the following case history:

> This is a quotation from the letter of a mother of a young boy who was a vaccine victim. "My son had a sore tailbone and was constipated. Tests showed that our 6 year old boy had 4th stage cancer and that he had less than a 15% chance of survival. The tumor occupied his whole rectum and he had metastases on his liver, lungs, and all the lymph nodes in his stomach. (We put him on) OregaRESP, Royal Power, Resvital, Purely-C, and GreensFlush. We gave him the oil of Oreganol. We started this right away, and he started taking it a week before chemotherapy. His protocol was 52 weeks of intense therapy, surgery, heavy radiation, bone marrow transplants, followed by more intense chemotherapy. He had (however) only 5 treatments (because) he was almost clear except for the spots on his liver...but they had decreased in size. They did a scan two months after surgery and there were a few spots remaining on his liver but they had decreased some more. I still wasn't interested in doing more chemo, so the doctor agreed to do (instead) another scan in two months—if the spots were still there we should start chemo again— and if not, then his (IV) line would come off and we would just monitor him. He had his scan (July 19, 2005) and he is completely cancer free. The spots on his liver are even gone. He took all of his natural medicines faithfully through his whole treatment. We thought maybe we could help others by telling it. I think that all of these natural products, along with God, saved my son's life.

Chapter 11
Medical Failure

Jonas Salk and Alfred Sabin did the human race a vast disservice. Rather than helping humanity they caused its decline. The infectious or AIDS epidemic may be largely the result of the original polio vaccines.

Because of their acts people suffer unmerciful pain and despair. Under the guise of saving humanity they accelerated its demise. The number of cancers directly caused by such men is legion. Uncountable people have been harmed; untold lives, certainly, hundreds of thousands, have been prematurely taken: all due to greed. Who were Salk and Sabin, and who supported them? Who created them into national icons? What's more, what was the real motive for foisting this agenda upon Westerners, this mass vaccination program using contaminated, in fact, carcinogenic, material? Who are the perpetrators, and what was their purpose? This because they have left uncountable victims in its wake, and the victimization is continuous, since this virus is readily spread through the generations.

Due to the deeds of a few men the brutality endured by the human race is beyond measure. Today, people endure unmerciful pain—the pain and agony of chronic disease and fulminant cancer—all due to the actions of the few.

The monkey manipulations were all for naught. This was no attempt to save humankind, nor did it have such an effect. The people who perpetrated this were either ignorant or devoid of the higher goals, that is of saving humanity. The fact is rather than help humanity it accelerated human decline. All scientists knew that monkey secretions were infective and that, in fact, they spread violent diseases. These diseases are so aggressive that they can lead to sudden death. There are untold millions of people who are infected with a wide range of monkey viruses.

For millions of such people these infections proved devastating. What's more, uncountable individuals have died from grotesque diseases, directly due to these infections and, therefore, the vaccination. What's more, as has been thoroughly documented simian virus infections are a primary cause of cancer.

This nation, the United States, bombs other nations, claiming to convert them to democracy. In foreign nations which it self-righteously deems a threat, it roasts people alive, blowing off body parts, killing wholesale, destroying entire cities, all supposedly for the sake of "freedom." Yet for its own citizens it is imposing an autocracy, forcing upon them deadly concoctions which create agony and disease. For Americans who are sick this has more to do with government policies; yet, billions of dollars of taxpayer money are spent in a nebulous war on terror, to supposedly prevent the citizens' harm. If the government is so worried about its citizens, why poison them with known carcinogenic viruses, which will assuredly give them cancers? Why intoxicate them with mercury, aspartame, and formaldehyde, all of which are proven carcinogens as well as neurotoxins? Is the creation of brain damage and cancer anything other than terror of the highest degree?

As a result of U.S. policies between 2003 and 2005 some 100,000 innocent people have been killed in Iraq alone. In the United States government policies have killed even more: some one million Americans from vaccine/drug poisoning. *JAMA* says that in the United States, yearly, nearly 120,000 people are killed by drugs, that is pills. MD Anderson notes that of the 55,000 people diagnosed with lymphoma yearly, some 60% suffer vaccine virus cancers. *JAMA* confirms that mutated germs, the result of the overuse of potent drugs, kill 250,000 yearly. The CDC notes that several thousand people yearly are poisoned or die from vaccine reactions, while the FDA describes that only a maximum of 10% of such reactions are reported. Regarding the drug-related deaths this fails to include the people who die in doctor's offices and/or shortly after an office visit. The majority of these numbers are gathered by hospitals. Thus, it becomes easy to determine that the estimate of one million deaths is low. Incredibly, the American people are victims of a kind of corporate-sponsored terror—the inflicting upon the people of death, despair, and disease, all for corporate profits.

Like all people Westerners are vulnerable to suggestion. The media attempts to train people how to think as well as react. Often, regarding terrorism people think of a nebulous concept, perhaps foreign invaders—dark-skinned Middle Easterners, "who don't like us." Without substantiation bizarre claims are made, for instance, "They hate us because of who we are and the freedom we represent." In contrast, Funk & Wagnall's definition of terrorism is entirely different. It claims that rather than an individual act it is a system, which is state sponsored, that is "The act of terrorizing (through) a *system of government* that seeks to *rule by intimidation.*"

It takes little to demonstrate the terror of this policy. This entire process was a waste. The people failed to benefit; the monkeys were tormented, drugged, brutalized, and slaughtered. Yet, all was for naught. This is because in order to eradicate polio no vaccine was necessary. Particularly, during the late

1950s and 1960s there was little to no risk for the general public contracting this disease. Why would millions of people be put at risk through the intake and/or injection of an animal serum, in some cases containing known live carcinogenic viruses, for a disease that was in decline?

Regarding the underlying cause of polio, particularly in the young, an early publication, *Practical Guide to Health*, is revealing. According to the authors the cause of infantile paralysis, that is polio, in infants and children, the pictures which so horrified and saddened the American public, is proven. It is contamination. It is a lack of sanitation. What's more, the direct carrier is the fly, in this case a special type known as the stable fly. This is an excellent book, with a self-description of "A Popular Treatise on Anatomy, Physiology, and Hygiene," with a "Scientific Description of Diseases, Their Causes and Treatment." It was written by F. M. Rossiter, M.D., a prominent member of the American Medical Association and superintendent of a major medical sanitarium. Rossiter was an expert in diseases of sanitation. Regarding polio he notes:

> The Massachusetts State Board of Health has very recently conducted experiments which prove that the stable fly has by its bite caused infantile paralysis (that is polio). This fly is different from the housefly. It is found in stables, and lives by biting animals, especially horses and cattle. It is not usually found in houses, but flies around in the sunshine. The stable fly is much more likely to bite than the housefly, and as it may enter the house before a storm, probably this is the fly that does the most of the biting of human beings.

> These discoveries go hand in hand with the fact that infantile paralysis (that is polio) is most common in the summertime or during the fly season....(polio) is most common in hot weather.

Romer, in his book, *Epidemic Infantile Paralysis*, confirms this. He clearly shows that in the United States, which was the primary epidemic site, virtually all outbreaks occurred during the summer. During that time in close proximity to humans there were hundreds of thousands of stables, as horses were still a major means of transportation. Horse blood contains various neurotropic viruses, and the biting flies could easily transmit these to humans. The gradual replacement of horses with automobiles was associated with a significant decline in the cases. The fact that this was a disease of pestilence is confirmed by the virtual absence of polio during the winter.

Charts provided by Romer demonstrate a spike in the cases during July and August, followed by a steady decline. In contrast, during the winter there were essentially no cases. The incidence during the coldest months is essentially nil, then, it gradually rises with the increasing temperature. For instance, during January the incidence was essentially zero. The same tendency was demonstrated in all other countries.

Universally, polio outbreaks occur only in hot weather. Romer was German, working in Marburg. The fact is this demonstrates that polio is caused by animal parasites. Incredibly, the cure surely cannot be to inject into humans such parasites. If it is a filth disease, then, rather than routinely injecting or orally dispensing more filth to people it is this which must be addressed. To inject animal contaminants—blood, serum, residues of urine, foreign protein, foreign DNA, residues of sperm, and other filth—would merely increase the vulnerability.

A curious finding was the virtual epidemic incidence of this primarily in America, during the war years. During the entire period of the polio epidemics America was at war, that is when the incidence was highest. The great epidemics occurred in 1943 through 1954, the latter date being the end of the Korean War.

Think about it. During the 1930s and 1940s polio was being extensively researched. This was an era when virtually any substance was considered fair game as a weapon. Why not a paralytic virus, perhaps sprayed from an airplane or pumped from a passing warship, all as an 'experiment' on the American or Canadian public? What better weapon for "fighting the enemy" than a virus, which would paralyze on exposure enemy soldiers or at least weaken them, making them a burden for their fellows. According to Judith Miller in her book, *Germs*, this is precisely what occurred, that is for various other organisms. This is far from a mere conspiracy claim. Documents uncovered via the Freedom of Information Act prove that in the late 1950s hundreds of thousands of Americans were exposed to a red-colored mist, sprayed towards American cities from warships. The contents: a biowarfare bacteria known as *Serratia marcesens*. The germ caused multiple cases of respiratory disease as well as a number of deaths. Thus, the purposeful release of paralytic germs into the environment is impossible to rule out. Nor can it be ruled out that, for instance, army horses were vaccinated with such viruses. Why else would there be such a wartime concentration of this disease? Another possibility is shedding, that is from vaccinated soldiers. Such contamination is plausible. Why else would America be the focus of this disease?

Yet, the real cause of the war-era spike remains unknown. Surely, another possibility is contamination from research, that is the 'escape' of the virus from research animals or infected humans, into the population. Plus, during the 1920s and 1930s the mutated virus was injected into various 'test' patients, and this could have led to its dissemination. It is well known that for even several months the virus can be shed from the infected, which can lead to the spread to others, even epidemics. Surely, residue from research—monkey blood, feces, and more—entered the waterways. Could children playing in waters downstream from the dumping site have contracted it in this manner? President Roosevelt himself is believed to have contracted polio from contaminated water.

Another possibility is changes in diet, which weaken the immune system. If the diet is poor, if it is high in starchy foods of low nutritional value, like bread, grits, and potatoes plus unhealthy meats, such as pork and dried/nitrated meat, then the outbreak of disease is likely. Furthermore, if it is high in sugar, this greatly depresses the immune system. The polio outbreaks were simultaneous with rather dramatic changes in the Western diet: the mass introduction of processed foods, which occurred primarily after World War II, precisely the time when polio reached its zenith. Prior to the introduction of such foods human beings were far healthier: degenerative diseases were essentially unknown. Suddenly, eating foods laced with food dyes, preservatives, white flour, refined sugar, hydrogenated oils, and nitrates became commonplace. As a result, the immune systems of Westerners were disrupted. Tonsillectomy also came in vogue, which also weakened resistance, since polio is an intestinal germ.

During the 1940s and 1950s astute physicians and chiropractic doctors noted that polio occurred more commonly in children addicted to sugar, therefore its association as the rich peoples' or 'suburban' disease. Rare among farm hands or country people, whose diets remained 'natural,' polio became almost exclusively a 'city' disease. This was also where many of the horse stables were found. The farmers, who continued to eat garden-fresh food and lived in a rather pure environment, were immune: the city people, who lived largely on processed foods and were exposed to poor sanitation, were vulnerable.

True, Rossiter notes the connection between the stable fly and paralytic polio. Obviously, this fly becomes infected by biting animals with the disease or through infected wastes, that is blood or sewage. Yet, he also notes that this fly usually bites its victims while trapped indoors and that this is where most transmission occurs. This coincides with the in-city outbreaks. Plus, the sugar-overloaded child is weakened and, therefore, vulnerable for systemic infection. In contrast, in the country people relied more on homegrown foods, which obviously kept them stronger.

The fact that outbreaks of polio are related to human wastes, that is fecal matter, is well established. Several outbreaks were traced to sewage-contaminated creeks, ponds, and swimming pools, where children were exposed. The fact is the polio virus is an enterovirus, meaning "within" or "intestinal." Thus, the primary source for outbreaks is sewage, particularly human sewage. If a society is completely sanitary, there will be no polio outbreaks. This further demonstrates the fraudulent nature of the vaccine.

Essentially, this is a non-communicable disease. It is not easily spread. This is an incredible finding, which fully debunks the vaccine claim. What's more, major outbreaks only occur in the summer, plus they usually occur in impoverished areas, where there is a lack of sanitation. Yet, poverty alone is insufficient as a cause. There are hundreds of cultures where there is proper sanitation, and even though the people are poor, there is no polio, unless such populations are vaccinated. Then, polio outbreaks occur. The fact is, today, in the Third World, as well as the Western world, vaccination is the number one cause of this disease.

Yet, the primary argument for vaccines is that they work—that they save humankind from the ravages of communicable diseases. Reports are provided to indicate that certain diseases were raging throughout humanity only to, after vaccination, suddenly plummet. McBean, in her book, *The Poisoned Needle*, proves otherwise. She provides a chart with the national cases of the major "vaccination" diseases before and after the introduction of inoculations. Incredibly, in the case of chickenpox, measles, German measles, and mumps, after the introduction of vaccinations the incidence of each of these diseases rose dramatically, in most cases more than doubling. So, in the Western world simultaneous with the introduction of inoculations such diseases were greatly declining. This indicates that vaccines were unnecessary and, what's more, since they contain the very disease-causing agents responsible for these ailments it only makes sense that the incidence would rise.

Medical authorities have only one objective: to protect their vested interests. Modern medicine is a monopoly, in which competition is brutally crushed. Drug reps have often told me as I attempt to disseminate this information that I am "dangerous." True, this information may be dangerous to certain individual's income but not to the general public. Rather, such information is clearly lifesaving.

Every year as a result of the evils of the medical system, tens of thousands, in fact, millions, of people are prematurely killed. Others writhe in agony and/or are maimed. Such deaths and disabilities are largely disguised. This explains Merck's infamous memo to its drug reps, saying that if doctors show concern about the deadly effects of its notorious killer drug, Vioxx, play "dodge ball Vioxx."

Over the past decade I have attempted to warn the general public about the dangers of certain drugs. While on the radio one drug rep countered me, saying, for instance, to call Vioxx a murderous drug was itself a "crime." How unfortunate it is, he complained, for the world to no longer to have this drug (a substance known to cause a minimum of 75,000 deaths), as he attempted to dissuade the public from my warnings, saying, "Now, without Vioxx what will happen *to the children*, who are in pain?" That is what Janet Reno said as she burned alive the children of Waco. Thus, again, government policies, as well as the arrogance of big business, are the main cause of human terror. This is certainly true of vaccinations, which cause a vast degree of human harm. Yet, it is little published, in other words, few people realize the enormous harm that these injections cause. A partial list of diseases caused by vaccinations includes:

lymphedema
lymphatic cancer
leukemia
brain cancer
intestinal cancer
bone cancer
colon cancer
lung cancer
wasting disease
muscle atrophy
multiple sclerosis
Lou Gehrig's disease
myasthenia gravis
multiple myeloma
pituitary tumor
epilepsy
attention deficit disorder
blindness or partial blindness
sudden infant death syndrome
juvenile arthritis
juvenile diabetes
eczema
psoriasis
chronic dermatitis
ankylosing spondylitis

spastic colitis
Crohn's disease
ulcerative colitis
malocclusion
TMJ syndrome
encephalitis
meningitis
Guillain Barré syndrome
lupus
rheumatoid arthritis
immune deficiency syndrome
sarcomas (Kaposi's, etc.)
chronic bronchitis
schizophrenia
Alzheimer's disease
Parkinson's disease
shingles
Bell's palsy
trigeminal neuralgia
impetigo
erysipelas
polio or polio-like syndromes
narcolepsy
neuritis
nephritis
pyelonephritis
neutropenia
autism
attention deficit disorder
hypogammaglobulinemia (low blood albumin levels)
hepatitis-like diseases
low blood albumin
testicular cancer

ovarian cancer
splenomegaly (enlarged spleen syndrome)
allergic shock
chronic allergies
chronic tonsillitis
Hashimoto's thyroiditis
hyperthyroidism
Addison's disease
adult-onset diabetes
Down's syndrome-like disorders
chronic fatigue syndrome
pericarditis (inflammation of the heart sac)
pleurisy
sudden death
inflammatory breast cancer
polymyositis rheumatica
irritable bowel syndrome
congestive heart failure
heart attacks
scoliosis
tuberculosis
pertussis

What an incredible list it is. Now it becomes apparent how truly destructive these injections are. The fact is this is a crime against humanity. Incredibly, some 70 diseases are listed. These are among the most frightening and agonizing diseases known. Yet modern vaccines are aimed at curing a mere 8 to 10 disorders. This makes it clear that rather than a cure they are the cause of human diseases.

How could any substance which causes such a vast array of diseases be a cure? The fact is this listing proves that vaccines are far from cures. Instead, they are disease-promoting. They are destructive to the human race, since they deplete the individual's vitality and immunity. Because of the toxic and microbial load that is injected into the body, they cause an inordinate degree of immune suppression. This makes the body highly vulnerable to attack, particularly by carcinogenic germs.

Early vaccine research proves this, that is that after vaccinations are given the immune system is drastically altered. Some investigators have determined a rather dramatic change in immunity happening quickly: within hours or days. There is never a positive benefit: only disruption and suppression. This makes sense. If toxins or germ components are introduced, rather than helping it this can only intoxicate the body. Merely for normal existence the human immune system is already under sufficient pressure. Why add to the burden through non-tested, in fact, toxic, injections?

It was J. W. Hodge, M.D., who had "considerable experience with vaccination," who as a result of that experience "denounced it." Then, after collecting his data he wrote the book, *The Vaccination Superstition*. In his book he claims:

> After a thorough investigation of the most authentic records (that is doctors' charts)...the conclusion is...instead of protecting its subjects from contagion...vaccine actually renders them more susceptible to it. Vaccination is the implantation of disease—that is its admitted purpose. Health is the ideal state to be sought, not disease...Every pathogenic disturbance (including the injection of vaccine toxins)...wastes and lowers vital powers, and thus diminishes its (resistance).

Even with smallpox, for which there has been continuous positive press about the benefits of vaccination, Hodge claims "after careful consideration of the history of vaccination...and after an experience derived from having vaccinated 3,000 subjects" that there is no proof that vaccination truly halts smallpox. More disturbingly, while emphasizing the logic of smallpox vaccinations he notes:

That the practice of vaccination has been the means of disseminating some of the most fatal and loathsome diseases.

That vaccination is not only useless, but positively injurious.

(That vaccination) depresses...natural resistance.

That immunity from all diseases is to be realized through the attainment of health, not by the propagation of disease.

That it is never necessary to set upon one disease in a healthy organism against another; that such a procedure is an appalling violation of the basic principles of hygiene and sanitary practice.

That (incredibly) smallpox epidemics invariably attack the vaccinated first.

That smallpox follows closely upon flagrant violations of the laws of health, hygiene and sanitation.

That...great epidemics of smallpox have coincided with periods of sanitary neglect.

That the community that has sanitary surroundings, a pure water supply, wholesome food, good health and freedom from the blood-poisoning effects of vaccination, need have no fear of smallpox or any other diseases.

This is a powerful demonstration of the fraud of vaccinations. His latter dictum is crucial: that in modern aseptic surroundings, combined with a healthy lifestyle, there is no need for such a treatment. Surely, in such a circumstance, the danger outweighs the benefit. Hodge describes vaccines as agents of blood-poisoning. If an organism is relatively pure, why poison it, for instance, a healthy baby? Yet, what is the definition of blood poisoning? It means that due to these injections a contaminant load has been added to the blood. The question is how could the addition of contaminants—toxic chemicals, such as mercury, aspartame, MSG, ethylene glycol, and formaldehyde as well as various pathogenic germs, as well as germ DNA—improve health? There could only be one consequence of such contamination: a decline in health.

The whatever-the-doctor-says concept is now dispelled. In other words, just because the medical profession promotes vaccines is no guarantee of effectiveness or safety. It was the medical profession which for decades instructed mothers to use aspirin, that is to suppress fevers. This resulted in the deaths of thousands of babies due to Reye's syndrome. In contrast, I never once prescribed it, knowing full well that fever was the natural means to kill germs and that repressing it would aggravate any disease. In Reye's the aspirin depressed the immune system, allowing viruses to run amok, destroying the brains of its victims.

Today, the medical profession continues its tyranny promoting unproven drugs, such as Celebrex, Bextra, and Vioxx, all of which have caused vast disability and fatality. Vioxx alone accounts for some 70,000 deaths in the United States alone, plus as many as 100,000 additional strokes and heart attacks: this is a minimum. This is an enormous degree of death and disability from a single drug—a drug which was known to kill long before it was removed from the market. One or two drugs kill more people than the entire American-Iraq war.

Yet, the entire vaccination concept is another example of failed trust. Even with smallpox vaccinations, the 'gold-standard' of preventive vaccination, there is suspicion of fraud. It was the wise Sir Clifford Albutt who said, "To mistake inferences or axioms for facts (that is to make an unproven issue as if fact) has been a curse of science." Albutt's prophetic words are confirmed by the fact that regarding smallpox "the most noticeable decrease...began with sanitation reforms just prior to 1800 and the improvements in nutrition brought about by health crusaders...(that is prior to such health crusaders the diet in America was poorly balanced)" What's more, the expansion of populations from the contaminated city centers to suburbia greatly reduced the incidence of communicable diseases, as did the establishment of regular garbage and proper sewage disposal. This had an immediate and provable effect on disease incidence.

During the early 1900s there were people living next to animals. There were various stables and pens, contaminated with wastes. All this was systematically cleansed, greatly reducing the risks for diseases of sanitation.

In fact, smallpox is readily spread by vaccination. This is particularly true for a hygienic society, where there is proper waste and sewage disposal as well as water purification. Statistics from vaccinations in England and Wales demonstrate the causative role of vaccinations in disease, notably smallpox. Early records show that when a campaign of mass vaccinations was instituted, including the mass vaccination of newborns, the incidence of smallpox dramatically increased. During the period 1872 to 1881, when some 97% of the parents submitted to this 'idea', some 3700 people died from smallpox. As a result, the reputation for compulsory vaccination suffered. For instance, in the period 1882 through 1891 the vaccination rate declined, while the death rate also declined to only 933. Then, from 1892 through 1901, when only 67% of the population submitted to the program, only 436 people died. This continued, until in the mid-1930s, when only 40% of the population was vaccinated and essentially no one died.

Obviously, the mass vaccination of infants proved deadly. What's more, clearly, the greater the percentage of people who are vaccinated the higher the death rate. Incredibly, like all other vaccines the smallpox inoculation is a fulminant killer, which disputes even the most remote possibility of any curative effect. Again, when mass vaccination for smallpox reaches nearly 100%, deaths from smallpox or smallpox-like diseases is high. Thus, in a society where methods of hygiene and sanitation are adequate, whether in the most remote regions of Africa or the modern cities of Europe, England, and America, rather than preventing it the introduction of any kind of smallpox vaccine, in fact, causes human devastation.

The government never seems to learn from its mistakes. Thus, in 2002 it introduced for smallpox a mass vaccination plan, primarily for health care workers as well as soldiers. There was no scientific basis put forth for the program: just that it was government-mandated. It was the *New England Journal of Medicine* (2002) which proclaimed that preventive mass vaccination of smallpox is medically inappropriate. Even so, in 2002 though 2003 the U.S. government foisted this vaccine upon the people, though they to a degree resisted it, vaccinating some 35,000 people. Of these, hundreds developed complications and dozens died.

The deaths were a kind of murder. This is because there was no medical reason, no medical indication, for the vaccination. Apparently, rather than a medical one the vaccination was based upon a business agenda. Yet, quickly, it became apparent that the vaccine was useless, and, thus, the program collapsed.

The cause of chronic disease?

In most people as a result of the inoculations the immune system never recovers. Thus, a chronic state of immune suppression develops. This may lead to a wide range of derangements, particularly chronic fatigue syndrome, fibromyalgia, polymyositis, eczema, psoriasis, and, ultimately, cancer. What's more, it would appear that vaccines are a conspiracy, that is the means to create disease and, therefore, business. Consider the trillions of dollars which are made from the treatment of the aforementioned diseases. Despite this it was L. Dublin, in his monograph, *Health Progress*, 1935-1945, presented by the Metropolitan Life Insurance Company, who said:

> ...the combined death rate of diphtheria, measles, scarlet fever, and whooping cough declined 95% among children ages 1 to 14 from 1911 to 1945, before the mass immunization programs started in the United States.

This is the ultimate proof against the deceptive nature of vaccines. Thus, it is only the most corrupt villains who promote such an agenda, which places the lives of untold millions of people, even babies and young children, at risk. What's more, if regardless of the cause the disease has been eradicated, why continue it? In the midst of such a massive decline in the incidence how could any credit be given to vaccines, that is for eradication? To give it credit and, in essence, fraudulently gain the trust of the people: this is tyranny.

It was social, cultural, and hygienic changes which were responsible for the vast decline in such diseases, not immunization. How could immunizations be credited? The fact is they cause disease. What's more, regarding such diseases this was a gradual, systematic decline, not a sudden obvious one post-vaccination. Regarding polio, as well as smallpox, the 95% reduction occurred without mass vaccination. This is evidence of the lack of any need for it. Thus, rather than mass vaccination it is more logical to conclude that the same factors which accounted for the original decline were responsible for any further decline. The vaccination programs were introduced during the plummeting of the curve. Thus, it is baseless to conclude that the vaccines are responsible. This has been the medical profession's argument all along, a most insecure one at that. The fact is it is mere disseminated propaganda unabashedly to maintain the power of the medical system, to perpetuate an attitude, that is of the submission of the American public.

In North America today ideal health is virtually unknown. This is largely due to the toxic effects of vaccinations, which have created a nation of biological cripples. If the people were vitally healthy, there would be no need for drug companies. There would be no need for the vast majority of medical machinery. Hospitals would be limited to trauma cases plus the care of the elderly and infirm. Chronic diseases would be significantly diminished, as would be cancers. The need for elective surgery would be minimized.

Vaccinations are a source of income, not for the mere cost of the vaccine but, rather, for the diseases they create. Here, again, some 60 different disease syndromes have been listed. These are virtually all new diseases. Thus, there are, in fact, diseases of vaccinations. These are diseases which were either non-existent or exceedingly rare prior to vaccinations. A list of the true vaccination diseases includes sarcomas, mesothelioma (a relatively rare type of lung cancer due specifically to simian virus 40), certain types of bone and brain cancer, certain types of eczema, certain cases of juvenile, that is Type 1, diabetes, mental retardation, attention deficit syndrome, autism, non-Hodgkin's lymphoma, certain types of leukemia, scleroderma, lupus-like diseases, eczema, juvenile rheumatoid arthritis, multiple sclerosis, Guillain Barré syndrome, and muscular dystrophy.

This is the true legacy of modern vaccinations. This is the result of the non-tested injection of gross materials with proven toxicity, including the highly poisonous merthiolate (that is thimerasol), formaldehyde, and numerous highly aggressive stealth germs.

The stealth germs are particularly dangerous. This is because as their name implies they fully evade immune surveillance. Thus, they readily infect the tissues, where they create the environment for tissue destruction. The fact is such stealth viruses are fully capable of creating chronic infections, which rapidly lead to cancer. Due to their toxic effects the immune system is fully disrupted, unable to cope with the infection: unable to even find the invader let alone destroy it. This is the type of biology that the vaccine makers inject into human beings. It is the biology of death, fully sanctioned by the governmental elite, many of whom profit handsomely from vaccine production.

It was Robert Bell, M.D., famous cancer specialist of the British Cancer Hospital, who said, "The chief, if not the sole, cause of this monstrous increase in cancer has been vaccination." This is surely attested to by the latest data, that is the direct connection of vaccine viruses with tumor development.

The vaccines are creating illnesses; they are not helping anyone. The challenge is can anyone prove that vaccines create good health and cause little if any harm? No one will take this challenge. Early American physicians apparently agree with this. S. S. Goldwater, M.D., New York's Commissioner of Hospitals, said in *Modern Hospital Magazine*:

> *The present measures used to check contagious diseases may permit a longer life—but not a stronger life. As a result of...vaccines...chronic diseases are growing at such a rate that America may become a nation of invalids.*

What a compelling statement it is. That vaccines have sapped the strength of this nation, robbing the people of their ultimate power, strong vital health, is irrefutable. The robust people who built America no longer exists. Vaccines have decimated the population. Rather than strengthening or protecting them, as people assumed, they denuded the peoples' immune systems. They imposed a burden that only the most monumental effort could reverse, such is the toxic load on the human body from vaccinations.

The greater the amount of vaccinations the individual receives the weaker the body becomes, and the more vulnerable it is to cancerous degeneration. This is because of the immense load of vaccine-induced toxins and germ agents, which contaminate the blood and internal organs. What's more, such toxins cause a kind of blood poisoning, which precedes cancer. Furthermore, as the immune system has been greatly weakened by the vaccines the various germ agents flourish. These germs cause cell damage, and, therefore, inflammation, leading to chronic infections and disease. The fact is such infections cause a vast degree of inflammation, which may lead to cancer. Says W. B. Clark regarding his direct observations:

> Cancer was practically unknown untold...(until) vaccination... I have had to do with 200 cases of cancer and I never saw a case of cancer in an unvaccinated person.

Dr. Clark's wise words were confirmed by another British investigator, Dr. Herbert Snow, Surgeon-in-Chief at London Cancer Hospital, who proclaimed:

> I am convinced that some 80 per cent of these cancer deaths are caused by the inoculations or vaccinations... These are well-known to cause grave and permanent disease of the heart also.

These are the words of one of Europe's top physicians regarding firsthand experience. Dr. Snow was able to directly tie the cases to the vaccinations. Again, it was Dr. Dennis Turnbull, who said:

> ...the most frequent disposing condition for cancerous development is...vaccination...

He also proclaimed that revaccination increases the risks for cancer cell growth. Thus, the highest risks for cancer are in those who have had numerous vaccinations, and those with the greatest numbers had the highest risks. In other words, incredibly, having only a few vaccines means a reduced cancer risk, while numerous vaccines means a high risk and large or repeated injections means a monumental risk. Dr. Turnbull was directly involved in the diagnosis and treatment of cancer cases caused by the vaccine.

In that era an entire book was published connecting cancer to vaccines, Esculapius' *Cancer and Vaccination*. Observers were acutely aware of the connection, because they saw first-hand the devastating effects of these serums. This was the first time that blood derivatives from animals were routinely injected into Americans, and, thus, novel diseases, which were previously unknown or were relatively rare, became epidemic. Says the author:

> ...an alarming increase in cancer is now evident. Those who adopt the brutal practice of calf-lymph vaccination are but too surely sowing...disease and national deterioration. Where the so-called human lymph is employed, syphilis, leprosy, and tuberculosis follow...and wherever calf-lymph is used, tuberculosis and cancer spread like a conflagration.

Note the mention of the use of human materials in vaccine manufacture. This is occurring today through the use of tissues from aborted fetuses. Syphilis is caused by spirochetes, which are wave-like bacteria capable of aggressively invading tissue. There are dozens of species of spirochetes, which cause syphilitic-like diseases. The syphilitic organisms may not cause genital syphilis per se, however, they may cause tissue destruction in a pattern similar to syphilis. It is this which afflicts many vaccine recipients, and this routinely evades medical evaluation.

Spirochetes are a kind of spore-forming bacteria. The spores are tough; thus, such organisms survive any sterilization procedures. The typical chemicals used in vaccines, formaldehyde and mercury, often fail to kill them, nor can these chemicals dissolve the spores.

This explains the case of Sheila S., who was the victim of an experimental vaccine: a new kind of DPT given to soldiers. Sheila, a national guardswoman, was a helicopter pilot. In the late 1980s she was immunized, only to suddenly experience a reaction. It was a syphilitic-like destruction of her facial bones as well as the bones and tissues of her sinus cavities and roof of her mouth.

Fully disfigured she was unable even to eat. To eat she plugged the hole that had developed in the roof of her mouth with bubble gum, so the food wouldn't go into the sinus cavities. Some 15 plastic surgeries and hundreds of drug prescriptions later she was no better. It was determined that she had sepsis of vaccine origin, to include syphilitic-like infections. She was placed on massive doses of wild oregano, notably the SuperStrength oil of wild oregano, the crude herb, that is the OregaMax, and the potent natural respiratory antibiotic, the OregaRESP (note: this is different than the OregaBiotic: it is for killing germs mainly in the sinuses, lungs, bronchii, etc.). This achieved something that some fifteen different antibiotics failed to accomplish: sterilization of the facial tissues. Now, she was able to undergo successful plastic surgery. As a result, her face, while disfigured, has been reconstructed, and she is now able to eat and function.

Sheila S. is an example of the types of catastrophes that occur but that are rarely recognized. While admitting that vaccine toxicity had caused her condition, her physicians failed to investigate it further to determine the real cause.

Why would the bones of this woman deteriorate, a perfectly healthy and vital American servicewoman? It could only be due to an active infection. The infection destroyed the cartilage of her nose, essentially consuming it. This is typical of syphilis. Incredibly, she became infected with a syphilitic germ, likely a contaminant of the animal tissues used to make the vaccine.

The source of the vaccine is unknown, although the possibilities include human fetal tissue, which could readily be infected with syphilis, monkey kidney tissue, mouse or dog cellular tissues, or, perhaps, cow or porcine cells. The making of vaccines is a filthy business. The vaccine companies realize it, yet, they foist their contaminated wares upon the public regardless.

Sheila's tissues are now healed, but only because of natural medicines. She now has healthy pink skin; her bones are partially reconstructed, as is her soft palate. The reconstructions are holding due to the eradication of the infection, including the heavily burrowed spirochetes. Thus, due to the powers of wild spice oils artificially induced syphilis, a vaccine catastrophe, has been cured. What's more, spirochetes are a major factor in tumors. This demonstrates the potentially cancerous effects of vaccine fluids. It was Dr. Benchetrit who stated that vaccines are largely "responsible for the increase of...cancer and heart disease," and the respected F. P. Millard, D. O., proclaimed that if vaccines were abolished, "the cancer death-rate" would be "cut in half." It is now known that cancer may be caused by syphilitic organisms. Vaccines introduce such organisms.

Cancer treatment is highly lucrative. This is one of the main reasons for maintaining, whether purposefully or subliminally, the vaccine agenda, since, surely, these injections (or pills, sugar cubes, syrups, etc.) are a greater factor in the creation of cancer than any other cause. Diet, while crucial, is not nearly as powerful as the injection of cancer-causing microbes and genetic material as a direct cause.

Yet, again it is the cancer consequences that are most devastating to humanity. What is most astounding is that these consequences are government-issue. Even more incredible is the fact that the epidemic could have largely been prevented by the most minimal government action.

There are those who would conclude that the government caused much of modern civilization's epidemics. To a large degree with cancer this is true. Janet Butel, M. D., director of molecular virology at Baylor College of Medicine, gives proof of this, when she proclaimed that one of the major types of cancers, lymphoma, is due largely to vaccine virus. Publishing in the *Lancet,* March 9th, 2002, she notes that "humans can be infected by SV40, an infection that was not suspected in the past" and that "this is an important finding because cancers with a viral cause (such as SV40-induced lymphoma)" could be 'theoretically prevented.'

The fact that vaccine viruses cause lymphoma is indisputable. Incredibly, this same issue of the *Lancet* contained a study by the University of Texas Southwestern's Dr. Adi Gazdar, who confirmed the presence of SV40 in non-Hodgkin's lymphomas.

Yet, the role played by various animal-derived drugs in the cause of cancer had long before been revealed. British investigators were particularly aware of this connection. An early writing by William Tebb, 1892, describes what was then regarded as a direct connection between the increase in cancer incidence and inoculations. Tebb begins by confirming that certain medical treatments become established in a virtual cult-like status.

Regardless of how much evidence is registered against them, he notes, the dogma is maintained as gospel. He calls the medical establishment the "orthodox medical church." Then, he proclaims that due to his concern for public health he will defy the system and present the true cause of the "remarkable and mysterious" increase in cancer during that era. He claims he was inspired to write his words as a result of seeing many of his friends and acquaintances die from the horrors of cancer, the origin of which none he could account for other than the forthcoming theory. Cancer, he notes, "is increasing at an alarming rate." In his book a chart is provided, demonstrating that in the mid-1800s cancer was exceedingly rare. In fifty years, that is by about 1890, the rate doubled. He then makes a compelling statement:

> Cancer is...increasing not only in England and the Continent (that is the European mainland), but in all parts of the world where vaccination is practiced.

It is well known that vaccinations cause blood poisoning. In that early era this was known as serum sickness, that is a toxic condition resulting from the injection of animal serums (another name for vaccinations). It was Sir James Piaget, one of England's most famous physicians, who said that cancer is due to a morbid condition of the blood, which, according to Tebb is largely physician-induced. This is because such a pre-cancerous condition can be caused by "impregnating the blood with impure matter." Dr. Joseph Jones, a famous American pathologist, observed that it is possible to create cancer through inoculation. In other words, in a body where there is no cancer, it can be gotten through injections. According to this pathologist, who studied post-mortem hundreds of cases, cancerous matter can be injected into the bloodstream, which will then cause cancerous growths. Dr. Von Bergman of Germany's Berlin Hospital reported in the *Medical Press* that cancer can be given to other humans through injections, including vaccines.

In the prestigious *British Medical Journal* a warning was issued that care must be taken in the exposure to even the tiniest amount of living tissue because it could transfer cancer. British legislators showed concern to such a degree that they reported the increase in cancer as directly due to contaminants in vaccines, including bizarre bacteria known as spirochetes.

Dennis Turnbull, M.D., a thirty-year cancer researcher, declared publically that vaccinations were the primary cause of cancer. Keurchenius, the former Colonial Secretary to the Holland Government, in public chambers noted the "alarming spread of cancer in the Netherlands, which was coincident with the spread of vaccination." In 1885 the *British Medical Journal* described in a leading article on cancer that the seed for this disease resulted from man-made contamination of cancer-causing germs directly into humans, notably the highly carcinogenic spirochetes, including the spirochetes which cause syphilis. It is notable in that era that human cells and lymph were used to make human inoculations, and such human material was routinely infected with cancer-causing agents.

Tebb quotes numerous early physicians, who, through careful clinical investigation, determined a direct connection with vaccines and cancer. They noted that the injection of animal-derived fluids led to infections which were unanticipated, including the introduction of syphilitic-like germs. These germs, known as spirochetes, are readily capable of causing tumors through spreading the "seeds of cancerous degeneration."

It was Herbert Snow, M.D., who called attention to the fact that cancer, while common in Westernized humans, is "Almost absent in (primitives)." Tebb notes that primitives resist any injections, refusing to allow their blood to be poisoned. Thus, such people escape the degeneration "under which cancerous tumors find nutriment." Then, describes Tebb, under the overpowering toxicity from the vaccinations, "The normal course of cancerous tumors (is a) steady increase, a steady and certain progress towards death." Thus, modern man has been bamboozled into accepting a fraud: that vaccines are a cure when, in fact, they are disease-causing. What's more, there is no long term benefit from modern vaccinations.

There has to be a reason for the rising incidence of this disease. There must also be an explanation for why the most dramatic increase has occurred since the mid-1950s. Yet, this was precisely the era for the initiation of mass vaccinations.

Chapter 12
Looming Disaster

There is a ticking time bomb afflicting Western man. Whether this internal bomb will explode is dependent upon a variety of factors. It is a race between the survival capacity of the individual—his or her genetic strength, lifestyle, and immune system—and the attempts of the invaders to overtake it.

In many people, particularly those who are under a great deal of stress or who are malnourished, the invaders win. SV40 and other monkey viruses are opportunists. They succeed in their viciousness only when the body fails, that is when it is no longer capable of fighting. When the fighting ability of the body is exhausted, only then does SV40 take over. Only then can it create the monstrous cancers it is capable of creating. Only then will it cause premature death.

There are exceptions. There are those whom it simply attacks and destroys. This occurs upon exposure to an exceptionally large dose. Yet, it is also due to vulnerability, a weakness, that allows it to succeed. To treat this disease every effort must be made to boost the immune system. This is no easy task. SV40 is a vigorous invader, highly elusive. It invades deep into the tissues, in fact, into the genetic matter. What's more, it operates via stealth. It becomes as if a part of the human genome, converting it to a substance, part human and part ape. This is the legacy created by the Salk and Sabin vaccines. Human bodies all over the world were contaminated with animal blood, testicular fluids, urine, and cells.

Scientists infer that "Science is God." The polio vaccine resulted in only human destruction. What's more, the destruction is continuous. Today, hundreds of millions of people suffer from weakened immunity, wasting diseases, exhaustion syndromes, autoimmune disorders, brain diseases, and cancer as a result of this 'unscientific' program.

The degree of terror this has caused is beyond comprehension. For instance, the vaccines are the direct cause of untold thousands, rather, millions, of deaths from cancer. With lymphoma alone there are some 55,000 cases per year. The majority of these are caused by vaccines, with the oral polio vaccine being the primary culprit.

The fact is the polio vaccine essentially caused this disease. The evidence is in the relatively low incidence of this disease prior to the vaccination. Since the 1940s the incidence of this disease has quadrupled.

The degree of devastation can be calculated. Since the vaccines were introduced in 1954 an estimate can be made. For instance, consider that there were on average world-wide some 100,000 cases of lymphoma per year since that time. This would place the total number of SV40-induced lymphoma cases at over 5 million. Then, there are a plethora of other cancers caused by this vicious agent, for instance, mesothelioma, bone cancer, inflammatory or infective breast cancer, prostate cancer, and brain cancer. The afflicted over this period, which spans some 50 years, amounts to additional millions. What's more, there is a suspicion that in some cases SV40 is the primary cause of leukemia. Plus, this virus has been directly implicated in various sarcomas. Even more ominous is the finding of SV40 in some 60% of any kind of newly diagnosed cancer. Thus, it is reasonable to presume that the Salk/Sabin fiasco is singlehandedly responsible for several million cases of cancer. This is the vile legacy of this vaccine, a gross public health disaster.

Any cancer which develops in an individual who was born from 1955 to 1964 is suspect of being due to SV40. Chemotherapy and radiation would fail to cure such cancers. However, the aggressive use of spice oils for destroying the causative viruses is potentially curative (see Appendix A).

Regarding the need for mass vaccination, such as the original national polio plan, as documented by a recent article in the *New England Journal of Medicine,* this is often overblown. According to the *Journal,* for instance, there is no medical need for mass vaccination against smallpox. What's more, repeated vaccinations grossly depress the immune system, increasing the individual's vulnerability to toxic diseases. For the individual who wishes to remain healthy the avoidance of modern vaccines is a must.

Natural medicine to the rescue

It is crucial for modern medicine to develop a new model. What's more, that model will be based upon the highest quality most effective natural medicines available. Here, the edible oil of wild oregano (P73) is invaluable, as are the highly potent multiple spice capsules known as OregaBiotic. These spice extracts are potent. The fact is they are capable of killing virtually any germ. The only germ tested thus far which was resistant was anthrax. Yet, everywhere it fully halted all growth, but it failed to completely kill it. The oil, as well as the OregaBiotic, effectively destroys entire categories of germs: bacteria, viruses, fungi, molds, yeasts, mites, and parasites.

Only through such a method will the health of Americans recover from the devastating effects of vaccine pathogens they suffer from modern medicine. Only then will they be able to, in fact, be protected from further catastrophes: all at the hands of man.

Scientific studies demonstrate that high potency edible spice extracts, notably oil of wild Oreganol (P73 blend) and the multiple spice complex, OregaBiotic, are capable of destroying a wide range of viruses. This is true even in the event of tissue viral infections, that is when the viruses deeply infect cells. According to an article accepted for publication by the journal *Antiviral Research,* P73 wild oregano oil eradicated virtually all traces of human cold and influenza viruses in a mere 20 minutes and this with only a single dose. Regarding the OregaBiotic, (a similar product is OregaRESP, also highly effective), this was even more destructive against the viruses tested, obliterating 100% of all human viruses in tissue culture plus some 99% of all bird (avian) flu viruses, again in less than 20 minutes. In general the OregaBiotic, which is a quadruple spice formula containing extracts of wild oregano, cumin, bay leaf, cinnamon, and sage, was some 25% more powerful than the oil. The OregaBiotic killed the viruses more quickly than the oil and also killed them more completely.

Yet, who needs treatment? Can it be determined if the individual is infected with SV40? This is relatively easy to ascertain. All that needs to be evaluated is: was the person injected with or exposed to the original contaminated vaccine? Did such a person take the oral polio sugar cube or syrup? Such individuals are fully contaminated with this virus, which now lives in virtually all cells of the body, including the brain. These vaccines were administered from 1954 through 1964. Then, there may be others who are contaminated who failed to receive this vaccine. There is evidence that even fairly recently, up to 1998, the vaccine was contaminated. The likelihood for such infection can be determined by taking the monkey virus symptom test on page 94.

There is hope for the individual chronically infected by stealth viruses, including SV40. A regimen of oil of wild Oreganol, plus the OregaBiotic, aids in the systematic eradication of this germ. For purging the system—the germ readily penetrates and grows in the brain and spinal cord—the wild oregano essence (that is the Juice of Oreganol) must also be added. For brain infections other aromatic essences may prove effective, such as essence of rosemary, sage, rose petals, and neroli orange. The protocol is as follows:

- oil of wild Oreganol (P73): ten or more drops twice daily. For tough conditions use the SuperStrength at the same dose.
- Wild oregano essence (Juice of Oreganol): one to two ounces daily. For tough conditions take two to four ounces daily.
- OregaBiotic (or OregaRESP): two capsules twice daily; for tough conditions take three capsules three times daily or even four capsules three times daily (always with food).
- Inflam-eez: an optional addition, helps fight inflammation throughout the body, making it easier for the body to heal: two or three capsules twice daily between meals.
- Neuroloft aromatic essences of rosemary, sage, and rose petals (a special formula for brain, mental, and spinal cord disorders): one ounce twice daily.

The aforementioned is the protocol which will purge the body of this devastating killer. Its purpose is to cleanse the body to the greatest degree possible of all traces of SV40 and similar simian viruses. The fact is in order for the sudden onset of disease to be prevented such viruses must be purged. The monkey virus is foreign to the body. If it is allowed to persist, it will likely cause cancer. It must be eradicated or the consequences will be dire. The only way to purge it is to use antiseptic spice oils, which are broad spectrum and can be taken in large doses. There is no toxicity in such extracts.

Vaccine makers have no regard for human life. This is obvious: formaldehyde is a known carcinogen, as is merthiolate, that is thimerasol. Yet, these are routinely injected into babies, children, teenagers, and adults. Is this anything other than absolute proof of the diabolical intent of the makers, who purposely increase the peoples' risks for degenerative diseases, including cancer? Both formaldehyde and thimerasol destroy human DNA, and so not only do they cause cancer but they also cause birth defects. Thus, tens of thousands of children now endure the endless agony of birth defects, including permanent brain damage, all because of the drug companies' greed.

The amoral nature of the cartel's approach is evident by the exposure of a recent experimental study on babies. Here, in highly ethnic regions of Los Angeles babies were injected with an experimental vaccine—without the parents' consent. This covert experiment did not occur in the 1940s but, rather, in the 1990s. According to the editors of the Web journal, *HealthSpring*:

> *Using kids as guinea pigs in potentially harmful vaccine experiments is every parent's worst nightmare. This actually happened in 1989 through 1991 when Kaiser Permanante of southern California and the US Centres for Disease Control (CDC) jointly conducted a measles vaccine experiment. Without...parental disclosure, the...vaccine (which, incidentally, was made in Yugoslavia)*

was tested on 1,500 poor, primarily black and Latino children in Los Angeles. Highly recommended by the World Health Organization (WHO), the high-potency experimental vaccine was previously injected into infants in Mexico, Haiti, and Africa. It was discontinued in these countries when it was discovered that children were dying in large numbers.

Thus, clearly, the purveyors of modern vaccines are evil, rather, they are fulminant murderers. Regarding the Los Angeles experiments the primary ill effect was chronic immunosuppression. Thus, the vaccine caused children with relatively healthy immune systems to become the victims of a chronically destabilized immune system, resulting in a wide range of disorders, including eczema, asthma, arthritis, ADD, chronic fatigue, and chronic infections.

As the scandal unfolded people demanded answers. In June 1996 the *Los Angeles Times*, producing a preemptive editorial, attempted to assure parents that, while such experiments were wrong, 'there is no evidence that any harm was done.' This is the typical protest, which the pharmaceutical cartel self-righteously disseminates: no evidence, no proof, utter denial. With such aggressive protesting, it can be presumed that there is much to hide.

From treating a single disease modern medicine created hundreds of others. Even if it were true that the vaccine eradicated polio, that it halted the progression of this crippling disease, yet, at what cost? S. C. Stenton writes in the *British Medical Journal*, March 21, 1998:

The introduction of the Salk...vaccine in the mid-1950s led to a drastic decline in the incidence of poliomyelitis (he fails to account for the fact that, independently, the incidence of polio was simultaneously plummeting, that is due to major improvements in sanitation). By 1961, the majority of young adults in Britain and American had been immunized and the numbers of reported cases of poliomyelitis had fallen from 8000 a year to 100 a year. At that point in the mass immunization programme, a contaminating virus was identified in the rhesus monkey kidney cells that were used to culture the poliovirus. It was named simian virus 40 (SV40). It was more resistant than poliovirus to chemical denaturation and survived...Early worries that the contaminant might be implicated in the development of human cancers have recently resurfaced. SV40...(has) a potent ability to induce tumors in species that are not their natural hosts...injection of SV40 into hamsters results in lymphoid tumors (that is lymphoma) and osteosarcoma (a kind of bone tumor).

What a poor exchange it is. Assuming Stenton is correct, the supposed eradication of a rapidly declining disease—all for brutal global cancer epidemic? Is the trade acceptable—8000 cases of a preventable disease versus, globally, some 250,000 or more cases yearly of lymphoma and untold other thousands of cases of bone, blood, lymphatic, breast, and lung cancers?

It is a vile consequence. Scientists create a global epidemic, while 'eradicating' another. Yet, consider the cost to this human race. The fact is the cost is unfathomable. The price paid by human lives—the loss of men and women, even tiny children and babies, before their time: this is a crime against humanity of the greatest degree. These scientists have created a horrifying legacy—for instance, it is the despair of the loss of a child or loved one—the agony of unmerciful unknown disease. This is the true legacy of the Salk/Sabin vaccines. It is the legacy of a devious government, which seeks to 'practice' medicine on an unwary yet trusting public. Is this anything other than the end of humankind? All it does is increase the costs of care, further bankrupting it. Vaccines are highly destructive. Rather than prevent disease they cause it.

To remain vitally healthy it is crucial to avoid being vaccinated. The less vaccine residues there are in the body the stronger will be the health. Compelling proof that vaccines are beneficial is lacking. On the contrary, there is a plethora of proof demonstrating their noxious effects.

As a rule children who fail to be vaccinated have a greater degree of vitality than the vaccinated. The fact is they have normal healthy immune systems. In contrast, those who are repeatedly vaccinated suffer from impaired immunity. What's more, the incidence of cancer in those free of vaccinations is significantly lower than in the vaccinated. Less cancer and degenerative disease, a reduced incidence in mental disorders, better behavior, a healthier heart, and a stronger immune system: these are the consequences of avoiding vaccination. The consequences of being vaccinated include a significantly higher risk for developing asthma, eczema, psoriasis, autoimmune diseases, chronic fatigue syndrome, arthritis, heart disease, stroke, cancer, and diabetes.

Vaccines can kill. It was Gary Null who reported a fairly recent vaccine-induced tragedy in Italy. In 1978 an experimental vaccine was given to a number of children, the diphtheria tetanus toxoid. According to Null:

> Within 24 hours, they were admitted to the hospital. Five of these children died and 59 additional deaths occurred within a period of eight months.

This is no accident. The fact is this is an atrocity. Yet, it is certain that the perpetrators failed to be held responsible for their crime. What's more, in addition to being poisonous and causing fatalities there is strong evidence that modern vaccinations fail to work, even for their slated purpose. Again, Null notes that since the introduction of mandatory pertussis vaccination, nationally, the pertussis rate has risen 3-fold. This is absolute proof that mass vaccination of a relatively healthy population is catastrophic. The fact is the vaccination created the very disease it was supposed to cure. This is another example of the amoral, in fact, evil, intent of the pharmaceutical cartel.

Null describes an even more obvious connection. The highest rate of vaccination in the United States, that is the greatest rate of compliance, was in 1993. Yet, this was also the year when the greatest number of cases of whooping cough, that is pertussis, occurred, some 5500 infected. That amounts to an epidemic, fully vaccine-induced.

It is not merely the pertussis vaccine that is fallacious. Marketed as a cure evidence exists that it too causes disease. This relates to other childhood vaccines such as the DPT (diptheria, pertussis, and tetanus) and MMR (measles, mumps, and rubella). A recent study evaluating overseas recipients of the MMR vaccine determined that recipients suffered a high incidence of allergies, twice that seen in those naturally exposed to measles. The investigators even postulated that instead of being harmful, developing the infection naturally bolstered the immune response, strengthening natural antibody production. What's more, it has been well established, for instance, by the work of C. Miller in the *British Medical Journal*, 1987, that the measles vaccine weakens the immune system. In this review it was found that regarding serious complications from measles vaccinated children fared worse than the people who had no vaccination. The fact is as a result of vaccinations the risks for measles-induced brain damage rose significantly.

Medical experts accept the fact that vaccines cause neurological damage. In the current medical literature the scope of the damage is impossible to quantify. This is largely because doctors grossly underreport vaccine-related side effects. The people are left to founder in their agony: the loss of a loved one, especially infants and young children, the despair of a brain-damaged or autistic child, the pain and fright of the development of juvenile diabetes. No, the fact is the vast majority of such sequela are never reported.

This is exemplified by a report on rubella immunization by Mitchell and his group in the *Archives of Internal Medicine.* Incredibly, the researchers note that a highly destructive side effect, sudden juvenile arthritis, is "uncommonly recognized" as being caused by vaccines and that, specifically, rubella vaccination, that is the MMR, causes "acute, recurrent, or persistent musculoskeletal manifestations." He describes two cases, both of whom shortly after vaccination developed joint pain throughout the body, arthritis, raised systemic rash, fever, numbness and tingling, and general weakness as well as pain, which persisted for years afterwards. Testing proved that the virus had contaminated the patients' white blood cells. The conclusion of the researchers was that in evaluating sudden onset of joint or muscular symptoms, especially in children or teenagers, 'rubella immunization or infection' must be considered. Yet, how rarely is it that doctors in the Western world ever consider this as a possible diagnosis?

Conclusion

The degree of devastation caused by vaccinations is so vast that it is beyond measure. Despite their destructive actions they continue to be dispensed. Yet, the diseases they are supposed to prevent are rising in incidence. It is curious that the decline of the health of native Africans is simultaneous with the introduction of modern vaccines.

Eventually, perhaps, researchers will sufficiently prove the destructive effects of these injections. Yet, clearly they cause more damage than good. The fact is they are a primary cause of disease and cause entire categories of novel syndromes. This demonstrates that the derogatory effects far outweigh the benefits. As people become more educated about the dangers of vaccinations less people will submit themselves or their children to these shots. This itself will be an interesting experiment. Will disease increase or decrease? Only time will tell.

There seems to be no limit regarding the tyranny which the drug companies inflict upon people: all for financial gain. A vaccine was proven to have the ability to cause cancer. It did so in all test animals. The vaccine could have been destroyed. Distribution could have been halted. Instead, the government released it. It had foreknowledge of the vaccine's carcinogenic actions. Yet, it enforced the campaign to dispense it. This is

300 The Cause for Cancer Revealed

fraud of the greatest degree: to use the citizens' monies, taken from them of their own good will, and use it against their interests and, then, incredibly, claim benefit. Rather than mere fraud this is vile tyranny of the most extreme degree.

Doctors and pharmacists tout the polio vaccine campaign as the ultimate proof of the greatness of modern medicine. This, they claim, is the true example, a proof that modern medicine is the savior. Modern medicine is the savior, rescuing humankind from medical perils, we are led to believe. Yet, is the polio shot the only example of an actual cure that medicine can attest to?

Even if it were true, how pitiful it is. There are some 80 years since the inception of modern medicine and is this all there is that can be claimed as a cure? In contrast, for hundreds of other diseases, including diabetes, arthritis, heart disease, lupus, and cancer, no cure is known. What a poor showing it is, because, incredibly, besides failing to cure any of these untold thousands of disorders it is, adding to the burden. This is because as a result of the barbarism of modern medicine numerous novel diseases have been created. In other words, incredibly, there are hundreds of man-made diseases, which are the result of medical and industrial corruption.

Medical companies and charities elicit donations and investments, however, the 'investors' gain no positive returns, rather, only misery. SV40 is certainly one of these human miseries, as is perhaps AIDS, *Serratia marcesens*, drug-resistant mutants, systemic candida infections, West Nile-like encephalitis, cancer, Lyme, chronic fatigue syndrome, polymyositis, ankylosing spondylitis, Guillain Barré syndrome, Gulf War syndrome, and fibromyalgia. Then, there are the drug-induced diseases: Steven-Johnson's syndrome, hives, eosinophilia, rhabdomyolitis (systemic destruction of muscle), aplastic anemia, and chemical hepatitis. The vaccine-induced diseases are pandemic: chronic fatigue syndrome, fibromyalgia, inflammation of the heart sac (pericarditis), autism, attention deficit, muscular dystrophy, myasthenia gravis, multiple sclerosis, ALS, Parkinson's disease, mental retardation, ankylosing spondylitis, juvenile rheumatoid arthritis, juvenile diabetes, leukemia, lymphoma, brain and bone cancers, Crohn's disease, and chronic bronchitis. These vaccines also cause in all ages sudden death. This is what modern medicine has produced. If it has as its only pride the cure of polio and smallpox, how truly pitiful is the effort. If this is all modern medicine has to offer, then, there is no real value to it.

This does not imply that all doctors and medical personnel are incompetent. Without doubt, in modern medicine there are numerous breakthroughs, primarily in the arenas of trauma or acute care. However, in chronic disease the medical offering is feeble if any. No cures are provided and, often, due to the treatment the disease process is aggravated. Premature death, in fact, fulminant medical catastrophes, are commonplace. People die at the hands of doctors and hospital staff. They die because of invasive treatments and drug therapy, even for rather innocuous conditions that would perhaps never solely cause death. For every life medicine saves, it would appear, it takes several.

Consider a mildly elevated cholesterol, joint inflammation, and perhaps, a slightly elevated blood pressure. All are treated with drugs, and every month, globally, thousands of people die in the Western world from the side effects of such drugs. These are people who died, rather, were killed, before their time. Thus, the pharmaceutical cartel is guilty of mass murder, that is of the very citizens who financially support it.

It is the public treasury which supports this corruption. This is what pays for the mass vaccination programs as well as the various drugs available through the government, that is Medicare and Medicaid. Think of the names: *Medi*-care, *Medi*-caid, in others words, government control of medicines. Rather, this system is merely the means to maintain the flow of money to the drug/chemical cartel, all mandated by so-called federal authority. The fact is the system is far from an aid, rather, it is a business for supporting the coffers of the drug and chemical companies. Indirectly, this also supports the oil conglomerate. Thus, in the Western government, there is seemingly no caring or aid. Rather, it is all about financial gain. What's more, the government is used as the tool, the reliable and oppressive means to gain access to the money. Contracts are dispensed by elected officials which favor the drug and chemical corporations of choice. Furthermore, whose money is it? It is the people's money. Is this anything other than fraud and racketeering? What a debacle it is that the public trust could be so fiercely violated, all in the name of personal greed.

This is also the story of the vaccine/drug cartel, with its six hundred-plus Capital Hill lobbyists. Rather than the medical profession the programs for mass vaccinations have always arisen from business interests. Thus, even the doctors are largely victims of this deception. If doctors have been involved, they have always been paid consultants, that is they are on the payroll of business interests. There has never occurred an altruistic mass vaccination program, done solely in the interests of public health. Proof for this is in the lack of effectiveness of most if not all mass vaccination programs.

Again, the DPT, specifically, the pertussis (P) component, is a good case in point. It was Gary Null who made clear in his article, *Vaccines: A Second Opinion,* the degree of the fraud. He quotes a study in the *New England Journal of Medicine*, 1994, describing an outbreak of pertussis in Cincinnati. Here, 80% of the children who contracted the disease had been fully or repeatedly vaccinated. The conclusion of the researchers was that since the children had been fully vaccinated, "it is clear that the...vaccine failed to give full protection against the disease."

He quotes other outbreaks, all in the vaccinated: 1997, Vermont, and 1996, Nova Scotia. Regarding the latter the outbreak occurred, despite the fact that nearly 95% of all children were vaccinated. He quotes another assessment, done by Birkebaek in *Clinical Infectious Diseases*, in which a telling discovery is made. It is that over "16% of individuals with chronic cough and no pulmonary disease were infected by B. pertussis." According to the researchers:

> Physicians should be aware of the impact of B. pertussis on coughing in adults, regardless of history of cough, because these patients may be a reservoir for B. pertussis and could potentially transmit the infection to infants, in whom the disease can be devastating.

In other words, the vaccinated, shedding or spewing their vaccine-induced germs, are causing epidemics in the population. They are acting as a brewery for germs, disseminating them, which may even lead to fatality. Thus, clearly, the DPT is no cure and, rather, it is the cause of disease, including the modern-day pertussis, that is whooping cough, epidemic. It was also Null, who wrote that since the "mandated pertussis vaccination in 1978, the incidence of the disease in the following eight years trebled...(and, incredibly,) While cases of pertussis were increasingly seen among every age group, the highest incidence was registered in infants less than 1 year of age...It is important to note that infants suffered from the most complications, with rates of hospitalization, pneumonia, convulsions, and encephalopathy (that is brain swelling and damage) being the highest in children 0 to 6 months old." Is this the legacy left by a supposedly preventive injection? The people in the Western world would be better off if no such vaccine was administered, that is if the DPT vaccine campaign was halted. The conclusion of the majority of the researchers is that rather than preventing pertussis the DPT is a major cause of the disease. Yet, incredibly, despite solid science proving its insufficiency, in fact, danger, the vaccine continues to be routinely administered to Western children. This demonstrates the tyrannical power of the medical system, where financial interests override the the needs and rights— even safety—of the people.

The effectiveness of vaccines has not been fully demonstrated. The fact is a number of these vaccination treatments have been proven virtually useless. Denver's Susan Dolan, R.N. and her group proved that the flu vaccine is of no consequence, and, now, as a result of the aforementioned research, it is apparent that the pertussis vaccine causes more harm than good.

It is well known that in children any vaccine can cause sudden death. Plus, the connection between modern childhood vaccinations and autism is irrefutable. Thus, vaccinations cause entire categories of diseases. This makes it clear that people today would be healthier if they avoid getting vaccinated than if they get vaccinated. Thus, of what consequence is such a therapy? If it fails to prevent disease, while, in fact, causing it, is there any reason to continue it? Is continuing such programs anything other than fraud, in fact, legalized murder? Plus, if there is even a slight risk of sudden death, why take it? In the United States a minimum of 10,000 people die every year from vaccine reactions. If the deaths from cancer are included, this number increases monumentally: some 100,000 yearly. These are mere minimums. This is far more than would die from the combined toxicity of all the diseases they are used to treat. Incredibly, financial interests are protected, while tens of millions people suffer and even die prematurely. Are corporate profits of such dire importance that human health, even human lives, are to be squandered, all for the sake of cash balances?

Vaccine makers offer no proof that their products save lives. All such claims are speculative. McBean notes that during the years 1880 to 1900 as a result of the introduction of sanitation and improved food supplies "the so-called contagious diseases declined...rapidly." Regarding these declining diseases none involved immunizations. Two diseases remained which failed to exponentially decline: smallpox and diphtheria. Yet, these were the very conditions for which vaccinations were routinely administered. Incredibly, she notes that during the late 1800s in dozens of hospitals the vast majority of the admissions for smallpox had a common parameter: all were vaccinated. Thus, during this era it was rare to see a person who failed to get vaccinated, who contracted the disease. This proves that for centuries vaccines have been foisted upon the public without evidence of cure. Surely, if they were a cure, they wouldn't cause diseases. What's more, there is little evidence that they truly protect the public.

Again, the British experience is revealing. In the late 1800s in Sheffield, England, where 97% of all inhabitants (some 200,000) had been repeatedly vaccinated, a smallpox epidemic struck the entire city, causing 648 deaths. Thus, it would appear the claim by the vaccine promoters for a smallpox, as well as polio, cure is baseless. Yet, even with all such facts held against it the vaccine industry keeps foisting its wares, insisting on a virtually almighty power, mandating that only through such a therapy can disease be "wiped out." Is the creation of entire new diseases, as well as multiple types of cancers—as well as the diseases in question themselves—is this synonymous with eradication?

It was Dr. H. M. Shelton who analyzed the true nature of the smallpox vaccination. This is critical, because it is upon the basis of this vaccination that medical professionals make their claims. Smallpox, they attest, one of the most fatal diseases of humankind, was singlehandedly eradicated because of vaccinations. This is why, they conclude, vaccinations are required. This is also the basis for condemning anyone who rejects vaccinations as a rebel. Yet, while vaccines may have helped save lives the fact is this method was a minor component compared to vast improvements in hygiene, sanitation, and nutrition. Says Shelton:

> I would not go so far as to say that vaccination has never saved (lives)...It is a matter of record that thousands of the victims of this superstitious rite have been saved from smallpox by the immunizing potency of death (that is the smallpox injections). But it is a fact that the official statistics of England and Wales show unmistakably that, while vaccination has killed ten times more people than smallpox, there has been a decrease in smallpox concomitant with the decrease in vaccination...(So), How could an operation that was declining be responsible for the extermination of smallpox?

Yet, to some authorities Shelton was too generous in giving vaccines credence. It was the early 20th century physician, Forbes Laurie, who said, *"vaccination contributes to the great increase in cancer."* An early governor of Maine, highly familiar with the vested interests of society, proclaimed that he had "grave doubts" about the effectiveness of vaccines and, what's more, that "commercialism exercised a considerable influence" upon vaccine policy. The famous Dr. W. H. Hay, author of a number of books, stated that there is "no proof of the boasted effectiveness of any form of...vaccine."

The English physician J. C. Ward, once a major proponent of vaccination, said the following after many years of experience:

> I believed that vaccination prevented smallpox. I believed that if it did not absolutely prevent it in every

case, it modified the disease in some cases, and also believed that re-vaccination, if only frequent enough, gave absolute immunity. Experience has driven all that out of my head; I have seen vaccinated persons get smallpox, and persons who had been vaccinated get smallpox, and I have seen those who had had smallpox get it a second time (because of the vaccination) and die of it.

What a crime against humanity it is, that is to convince the population of the value of a procedure which offers the opposite: only agonizing pain. Yet, Ward's exposition is compelling, because he was a vaccine proponent, an orthodox medical doctor, who after direct experience found the entire system a fraud. It is proof that untold millions have been deceived, and that for modern society vaccines are unnecessary. Yet, considering Ward's words literally, even the 'gold standard' of medical vaccination—the key for all success claims—the eradication of smallpox and polio—is based upon deceit.

Ward, who had direct experience with the most highly touted vaccine known, the smallpox inoculation, stated a simple fact: that the vaccine caused far more death and despair than any benefit. This is a firsthand account, which is far more credible than the proclamations of today's experts and physicians, who seek to promote the value of their profession. Ward saw precisely the consequences of mass vaccination and concluded that there was far more harm than benefit.

The degree of destruction perpetrated by the vaccinations is beyond comprehension. This is again demonstrated by first-hand accounts. For instance, consider the observations of Dr. Walter M. James of Philadelphia. Incredibly, this physician directly connected the early 20th century outbreaks of TB with vaccinations. He also documented numerous cases of cancer directly due to inoculations. He clearly observed that such injections foisted upon the unsuspecting public caused fatal diseases, tracing the cancer epidemic to such inoculations. Thus, he too concluded that the harm exceeded the benefit.

It is important to realize that this is far from an ancient problem. Today, in the Western world, as well as Third World, vaccine poisoning is occurring. Peoples' immune systems are being systematically destroyed, all due to the overload created by the inoculations. New diseases are being introduced. Immunity is being artificially altered. The vulnerability of the population is being increased.

Is this synonymous with preventive medicine? The fact is as a result of mass vaccinations greater amounts of medicines are required merely to treat the crippling side effects which result from these injections. Vaccination victims develop a wide range of chronic, even bizarre, diseases, and, thus, seek medical care. Then, they are often placed upon multiple drugs. Thus, vaccinations are "good for business." In contrast, people who avoid vaccinations are healthier than those who are heavily vaccinated. What's more, they require little if any medicine. Plus, they live a longer and more vital life.

This reveals a potential for conspiracy, that is the conspiracy of creating disease to further corporate profits. When a man of the stature of J. Anthony Morris, Chief Virologist of the federal government, made such a claim, that is that the vaccines are harmful, as well as useless, and, yet, they are forced upon us regardless, can there be any other conclusion?

The vaccine viruses are in the tissues of the children, even today's children—even newborns. They are within the tissues of the elderly and infirm, the strong and powerful, the young and vigorous, the weak and the tired. The fact is the population has been fully contaminated. Regarding this there can be no doubt. Entire lives have been destroyed, all due to the greed of a few arrogant politicians, industrialists, and scientists.

Now, there is an epidemic, which is entirely man-made. People have been injected with or exposed to a fulminant cancer-causing virus. It is a virus of such virulence that it causes cancer in every animal which receives it. Surely, it is the most prominent cause of human cancers known.

There is little which can be determined as a true cause of cancer. In contrast, SV40 and associated simian viruses are irrefutable causes. They simply cause cancer where it would otherwise fail to occur. This is absolute proof of the murderous effects of human greed. Surely, the perpetrators must be held accountable.

During the 1950s and 1960s it was Bernice Eddy, whose lab tests demonstrated the presence of a cancer-causing virus, in fact, SV40 and its relatives, in the human vaccine. When she warned authorities, her company was closed. A scandal erupted, leading to a U.S. Senate investigation: Eddy's data was fully revealed, when she warned legislators that "unless the vaccine contamination problem was addressed, slow monkey viruses would create *cancer pandemics globally*."

Eddy was proven prophetic. Clearly, the virus is found within Westerners, particularly Americans. Here, unless it is purged from the tissues, it will surely cause cancer. It was the University of Southern California's W. J. Martin, M.D., Ph.D., one of the world's top pathologists and immunologists, who made the connection. He found bizarre vaccine viruses, traced to the original monkey tissues upon which they are grown, to cause diseases in both adults and children.

The diseases associated with monkey-source vaccines, the slow viruses of Dr. Eddy, include autism, attention deficit disorder, muscular dystrophy, myasthenia gravis, Alzheimer's disease, Parkinson's disease, ALS, MS, chronic fatigue syndrome, fibromyalgia, autoimmune disorders, depression, schizophrenia, anxiety, seizures, developmental delays, asthma, mental retardation, lupus, cerebral palsy, and encephalitis.

Ominously, modern research is proving Dr. Eddy to be correct. It was again W.J. Martin at his Infectious Diseases and Molecular Pathology Laboratories who made the discovery. According to Thomas Stone, M.D., Martin had been "meticulously culturing out stealth viruses from patients for…years and, in a stunning development…successfully identified one of the viruses as being of African green monkey origin by using DNA sequence analysis." Yet, in what is a little-known revelation the fact is the risk for contamination is modern. During the last three decades kidney tissues from African green monkeys have been used to make the live oral polio vaccine as well as other viral vaccines. Thus, this human race is infected to a degree beyond comprehension. Especially in the Western world if there is a chronic disease, cause unknown, it is likely due to such stealth viruses, which consistently degrade health and which, if left uncontested, cause the individual's premature demise.

Vaccine viruses must be purged. This can only be achieved through potent natural germicides, that is the wild spice oils/extracts. OregaBiotic, the wild sage, oregano, and cumin extract, is ideal for this, as is the P73 oil of wild oregano. These are potent germicides capable of eradicating such viruses. OregaBiotic aggressively purges this virus from the system. The wild oregano steam essence, that is the Juice of Oregano, is also critical. This is because it is water soluble and, therefore, crosses the blood-brain barrier. Neuroloft is also invaluable and may aid in nerve cell regeneration. This is a combination of spice essences including essences of sage, rosemary, rose, and orange blossom. It also crosses the blood-brain barrier. There is also the OregaSpray, which is an effective barrier to prevent infection as well as to topically destroy germs. What's more, black seed is also antiviral, especially oil of black seed.

For ultimate success the liver must also be purged. This can be accomplished through spice extract capsules plus a kind of herbal flush, which stimulates bile flow (see Appendix A). Here too oil of black seed is also effective as well as a wild greens extract, that is GreensFlush.

Aromatic spice therapy is the only truly reliable means to treat this condition. However, in extreme cases it may take a considerable amount of time, such as six months or a year, perhaps two years, to purge this organism from the tissues.

The government and greedy businessmen created this disease, and the natural substances cure it. In particular, oil of wild oregano (P73), as well as multiple spice capsules containing garlic and onion, the OregaBiotic, are capable of purging this agent from the tissues. Again, the pharmaceutical houses created the disease, while the divine or natural powers reverse it.

The health of the immune system is also inhanced by the removal of heavy metals. The GreensFlush and for the kidneys the CranFlush (see Appendix A) are useful in this regard, as is the GrapeFast. The latter is a wild grape extract rich in tartaric acid, a powerful agent for purging heavy metals. All such extracts also cleanse the liver, as well as kidneys, increasing the body's resistance against disease. To order these wild medicines check superior health food stores or call 1-800-243-5242. The combination of the Greens/CranFlush plus the wild grape extract GrapeFast will mobilize and cleanse heavy metals from the body. Then, there will be a major improvement in health, and the risks for SV40- and stealth virus-induced diseases will be dramatically reduced. The only way to fully minimize the risks is to routinely take the wild spice extracts, that is on a daily or maintenance basis. The maintenance amount varies from one or two OregaBiotic capsules daily, and the oil, three to ten drops twice daily. The Juice should also be taken as a maintenance, two tablespoons daily.

This is a major endeavor, that is to eradicate such viruses. Yet, with a conscientious effort it can be achieved. The protocol for this therapy is found in Appendix A. It consists of the intake of oil of wild oregano, ideally sublingually, OregaBiotic, wild oregano essence, that is the Juice of Oregano, and the cold-pressed garlic extract, that is the Garlex. Regarding the latter it is primarily a lymphatic cleanser. However, it is also a natural germicide and is particularly effective against yeasts and parasites. This is the purge that will prove lifesaving, particularly in relation to the prevention of potentially fatal diseases such as cancer, heart disease, stroke, and diabetes.

For most Westerners with cronic diseases the diagnosis of SV40 and similar stealth viruses must be presumed. The symptom test is included in this book. This is the most accurate way to determine the existence of the infection. There is no common blood test for this disease.

SV40 was preventable. Researchers, as well as the government, were well aware of the contamination. The mass vaccination program could have been halted, but, instead, financial concerns took precedent. Is it that the people of this Earth no longer care for their fellow men? Certainly, this is true of the purveyors of modern medicine, particularly the vaccine and drug manufacturers. Today, deaths due to drug and vaccination toxicity number in the millions every year. In the United States alone some 500,000 people die from drug or vaccine reactions/toxicity, making this virtually the primary cause of death, perhaps only exceeded by cancer.

People fail to realize that vaccines are drugs. They are merely the injectable form. Mercury is a drug, as is, perhaps, formaldehyde. Drugs are defined as cellular poisons. How could a cellular poison aid health? How could it boost or normalize immunity? How could it prevent or cure disease? Yet, people are under the impression that vaccines achieve precisely this. The fact is such thinking is grossly flawed.

The divine being has provided on this earth all that is necessary to heal the body. Scientists are now certain that rather than the result of spontaneous evolution the human body results from a Creative Power. Natural medicines made by that same Creative Power simply work better, while infinitely safer than the man-made. Thus, natural substances can be relied upon to cure common diseases, including the so-called vaccination diseases. Healthy doses of spice extracts, propolis extracts, garlic, onion, and natural vitamin C are all that is needed to ward off such supposed killers. There is no need to fear the vaccine diseases. The fact is this fear has been created by the very industry which profits from it. Measles, mumps, chicken pox, and rubella: all are thoroughly destroyed by spice extracts. Furthermore, a greater number of people die as a result of vaccine therapy than any such diseases.

Through the regular intake of herbal or spice-based formulas the immune system is strengthened. To prevent any such illness or any of the complications this is all that is required.

Yet, the key with natural substances is the potency. It is necessary to use formulas which produce results. Such formulas must also be free of contaminants. It is also crucial to know which foods and formulae have a scientific basis for their effects. This can be achieved by the individual's own effort: by contacting the company to ensure that there is science and that there is a sound basis for the formula. With the wild oregano extracts there is unprecedented proof that, in fact, such extracts are effective. The same is true of other key substances mentioned in this book: propolis, raw honey, natural-source vitamin C, cumin, sage, cinnamon, wild greens extracts, and garlic. All such substances have a plethora of scientific studies to support any claims.

The science regarding oregano extracts is perhaps most compelling. Here, only the P73 extract has been shown to be effective, as well as safe, both in test-tube studies and in humans. In humans studies using the P73 have proven that even in large amounts dozens or even hundreds of drops daily, are fully safe and free of any organ toxicity. The P73 material is made from the wild-growing mountain spice.

With the P73 and similar spice oils (North American Herb & Spice) only steam is used for extraction. Thus, it is highly pure, free of any chemicals. Beware of cheap imitations, which have no scientific basis and which, in fact, may be harmful. In one instance, false or inexpensive oregano oil caused the death of a dog. In contrast, some 2 million North Americans use the P73, without even the slightest untoward effects. Thus, it is highly safe, free of any human or animal danger. In fact, this extract is commonly used by exotic bird owners, as well as pet shops, to prevent respiratory ailments in their birds. In one instance an exotic bird expert saved dozens of tropical birds merely by adding the P73 oil of oregano to the drinking water. This fully demonstrates that drugs are overused, while the potential of nutrients, spice extracts, and herbs is untapped.

People have been poisoned due to their own lack of knowledge. It is also their vulnerability to fear that is responsible. People are afraid to die; they will do all that is necessary to avoid it. People who hold to a higher belief, who accept the ultimate return, who realize the reality of the transition, are less likely to fall prey to such fears. Thus, such individuals can more rationally evaluate their health challenges without succumbing to the fear tactics of doctors.

People believe that undergoing invasive treatments or taking numerous medications will forestall death. Yet, recent reports demonstrate the highly fatal effects of various surgeries and drugs. From the glaring statistics of drug-related deaths and disease it is obvious that such substances fail to heal disease. In the hospital or pharmacy, incredibly, there are few if any cures.

Before taking any drug, including inoculations, be sure there is a sound basis for it. This is because with drug therapy the risk for sudden death, as well as organ damage, is high. This is far from fear tactics: a minimum of 500,000 deaths due to drugs and vaccines is surely sufficient proof of the danger of pharmaceutical agents. Rather, it is lifesaving and fear-preventing: to become informed about the risks rather than blindly trusting in the 'system.' The fact is the agents themselves have proven their status—due to their unbridled greed the companies are causing their own destruction. According to FDA sources one drug alone, Vioxx, is responsible for a minimum of 85,000 deaths.

If the pharmaceutical cartel falls into public disfavor, it will destroy itself. People will fail to trust any of its proclamations. There will be a general distrust of its motives, even its science. When the drug rep pitches his/her wares, it will be regarded with a jaundiced eye. This will be the cartel's own doing. The "Dodge-Ball Vioxx" memo has proven that.

That human beings could, under the guise of 'prevention' or 'cure' kill other humans, while fully disguising it, demonstrates the depravity to which humankind has descended. For every drug pharmaceutical companies accept a certain number of deaths. What's more, they show no remorse. The fact is they cover up any evidence for the destruction they cause. Furthermore, they earn the favor of public officials, essentially bribing them, to position themselves.

Where do they get the money for such bribes? It is from the public coffers, since they derive much of their profits from government contracts. In other words, they purge the public treasury and use these profits to flog their productions. It is a vicious cycle, with the drug companies and elected officials working in unison to earn major income, while victimizing the public. The fact is the public fails to gain in any way from this method. Officials are given special gifts, trips for the family, and contracts in the name of, perhaps, distant relatives: all so that there is no 'obvious' connection. Then, the officials, whose favor has been earned or, rather, bribed, ease restrictions, bringing potentially fatal drugs into the market. From the public treasury they award multi-million dollar contracts to help establish the drugs. The fact is drug companies desire easy income: large government contracts, that is tax dollars.

The corruption in medicine must be halted. No one should be forced to endure a poisonous therapy. Special interest groups must be eliminated. Corrupt officials must be sacked. Programs based upon merely financial gain with utter disregard of the needs and rights of the people must be purged. People must no longer be used as mere experiments, with no regard to their inalienable rights.

The blatant harm of the fellow man for mere selfish gain must be halted. Otherwise, there is no chance of humanity's survival. Nor is there any future for this planet Earth. If corruption is allowed to hold sway, humankind will descend into chaos. Only raw tyranny will rule. All will be lost. It will be the end of civilization as we know it. This has already happened: much of humanity suffers the consequences of the vile SV40, a creation of lust and greed. Thus, rather than an act of God it will be humankind's own wickedness which will destroy it. Now, millions of people suffer in utter agony. What's more, countless have died prematurely. SV40 is responsible for unmeasurable cases of cancer. It also causes vast numbers of other syndromes, particularly neurological and inflammatory diseases. It also causes immune deficiency. Neurological disorders caused by SV40 include multiple sclerosis, ALS, Parkinson's disease, seizure syndromes, and Alzheimer's disease. Yet, its role in cancer is diabolical. The fact is the polio vaccine and its vaccine contaminants are perhaps the number one cause of cancer in the modern world. To reduce the cancer risk the vaccine virus must be purged, (see page 324 for protocol).

Appendix A

Dietary recommendations: the ideal diet for reversal of stealth viral infections

Fatty acids are antiviral. They are the most antiseptic of all foods. Plus, they stimulate the flow of bile, itself an antiseptic. What's more, fat stimulates the absorption of spice oils, helping deliver them to the blood and lymph. In the stealth virus purge a high amount of natural fats should be consumed.

Certainly, natural vegetable fats are a focus of this diet. However, so are animal fats. This is because animal fats help nourish the cells with vital compounds unavailable in vegetables. What's more, they provide cholesterol, which is crucial for the protection of cells. Plus, animal fats are the richest sources of the crucial fat soluble vitamins A and D, both of which are needed for strong immunity.

Animal fats greatly increase the flow of bile. The bile helps purge the liver of harmful germs as well as toxins. Without it, the liver stagnates, leading to gallstones as well as infection. A stagnant liver greatly impairs the ability of the body to heal. In order to successfully eliminate any virus the liver must be active in its secretions. This requires the regular intake of fatty foods. Even if animal foods are restricted, at a minimum natural healthy vegetable fats must be regularly consumed, such as extra virgin olive oil, nut butters, nuts, seeds, red palm oil, black seed oil, and avocados. This will help maintain the flow of bile. Essentially fatty acids are also antiviral. They protect the cells against cancerous invasions. Here, a berry seed essentially fatty acid supplement is ideal, that is EFA Orega.

Regarding the low-fat diet a common consequence is degeneration of the liver and gallbladder. What's more, with such a diet there is a significant increase in the incidence of gallstones, in fact, the low-fat diet is a primary cause of this condition. When the synthesis of biliary juices declines or ceases, as occurs on a strict low-fat diet, as well as in most vegan diets, this leads to localized infection. In other words, the gallbladder and liver will become infested with germs. This makes sense: if there is a halt in the flow of fluids, then, just as in a stagnant pool of water, there is teeming infection, that is versus the rather germ-free flowing stream. The same will occur in the liver and gallbladder. Thus, the steady flow of bile helps prevent the development of liver and intestinal infections.

This is critical, because, in order to fully purge the body of stealth viruses the support of the liver is required. The liver contains untold millions of specialized cells, which cleanse the blood of all toxins, and this includes dangerous germs. These cells are known as Kuppfer cells, and they are particularly situated in the liver for trapping any invaders. Bile nourishes these cells; without it they die. Thus, on a daily basis it is crucial to maintain the intake of natural fats. Thus, the low-fat diet is destructive in regards to these organs.

A high animal food diet aids in the recovery from this disease. This is largely because of the rich amounts of liver-stimulating fats in such foods, but it is also a result of the high content of vitamins A and D, both of which strengthen immunity. It is also because animal foods are a rich source of amino acids, which are needed for cellular repair. The amino acids are also the essential component for cell synthesis, for instance, the synthesis of white blood cells and immunoglobulins. Plus, animal foods are rich in essential amino acids. These amino acids are needed for immune cell synthesis as well as tissue repair. For the treatment of SV40 infection do not follow a vegetable/fruit only vegan diet.

This is no license to dine excessively, that is on huge steaks and chops. Only the most healthy and pure animal food sources are allowed. This means exclusively organic or grass-fed animal sources. Again, the animal protein provides amino acids, direly needed by the immune system. Plus, animal foods are rich in certain key vitamins, notably vitamin A, vitamin D, riboflavin, and pantothenic acid, which bolster immunity and aid in the eradication of the virus. Amino acids are antiviral. This is why animal foods are a crucial part of the diet.

Only the organs and skin contain vitamins A and D. The exception is fatty fish, where it is found in the flesh. Milk and eggs also contain a fair amount. These foods are also high in fuel components, various fatty acids, lecithin, cholesterol, palmitic acid, carnitine, and taurine, all of which aid cellular metabolism. None of such substances can be procured through eating vegetable foods. Again, these vitamins are needed for this optimal antiviral defense.

The following foods are ideal for this diet:

Animal foods (organic/grass-fed)

whole milk
whole milk cheeses
kefir
kefir cheese
beef
bison

yogurt
quark
whole chicken eggs
whole duck eggs
quail eggs
turkey

venison

elk

quail

goose

duck

Fish and seafood

Note: beware of the elevated mercury levels in large fish

sardines

herring

cod

whitefish

halibut

shrimp

mahi mahi

tilapia

crab

red snapper

grouper

salmon

lobster

trout

arctic char

Vegetables

eggplant

green string beans

yellow wax beans

green and red peppers

Brussels sprouts

onions

leeks

radishes

watercress

romaine lettuce

red leaf lettuce

squash of all types

kale

kohlrabi

broccoli

cauliflower

cabbage

garlic

turnips

horseradish

arugula

bibb lettuce

beets

zucchini

Fruit (low sugar; excessive amounts of sugar depress immunity)

oranges
grapefruit
lemon
pomegranate
papaya
star fruit

tomatoes
avocados
lime
strawberries
kiwi

strawberries (due to heavy pesticide contamination only consume organic)

berries of all kinds, especially currants and cranberries

Carbohydrates/starches

baked potato with skin
amaranth
lentils
garbanzo beans

wild rice
brown rice
quinoa

Nuts and seeds

This should be limited to Brazil nuts, pumpkin seeds, almonds, filberts, pistachios, and sunflower seeds (no cashews, peanuts, or peanut butter).

Condiments

horseradish paste
sea salt
olives
extra virgin olive oil
sesame paste (tahini)
unsweetened ketchup (Unketchup)
raw crude honey (where bees are not fed sugar)
coconut oil (that is the spice-infused CocaPalm)

vinegar
mustard
kelp/seaweed
sesame oil (Sesam-E)
spices

Food to strictly avoid:

All beans and legumes, except garbanzos and lentils must be avoided. Beans are high in arginine, which fuels viral growth. No peanut products of any kind must be eaten. Nuts, such as pecans, filberts, walnuts, Brazil nuts, and almonds, may be eaten but not as the main source of protein. Rather, animal foods should be the preferred protein source. There should be an emphasis on organic milk/yogurt and wild fatty fish. Wild game and/or bison would be preferable to beef, although organic beef is a healthy food. Such foods are rich in the viral antagonist, lysine. What's more, no chocolate of any kind can be consumed. This is because chocolate is exceptionally rich in arginine, which accelerates the growth of viruses.

All alcohol beverages must be avoided, including red wine. Alcohol destroys the intestinal lining. This increases the risks for dangerous infections. What's more, the regular intake of alcohol leads to bone marrow damage, which direly impacts immune function.

Note: All foods not on this list should be avoided. The intake of processed and fast foods should be curtailed.

List of products mentioned in this book

- CocaPalm (a high grade extra virgin coconut and red palm oil cooking and spreading oil infused with wild spice oils; this is the ideal cooking fat)
- Oreganol oil of wild oregano (P73)
- CranFlush
- GreensFlush wild greens formula
- GrapeFast wild grape extract
- Inflam-eez
- Oil of Propolis (PropaHeal)

- Thyroset (formerly ThyroKelp)
- Royal Power (formerly Royal Kick)
- OregaMax
- Juice of wild Oregano (Oreganol P73 juice)
- Kid-e-Kare rubbing oil, gelcaps, antiseptic/wild cherry throat spray
- Germ-a-Clenz essential spice oil spray
- Sesam-E
- Oil of Black Seed
- Neuroloft Essence
- Pumpkinol
- EFA Orega
- CocaPalm (this oil for cooking is antiviral)

All such products are made by North American Herb & Spice. All provide antiseptic, antibiotic, cleansing, and antiinflammatory powers. Plus, such products support the health of the cells and glands, while helping cleanse the body of toxins. To buy such products request them from high quality health food stores. Also check the internet site (P-73.com) or call 1-800-243-5242.

With effort, the products can be found. These are high-quality products made from completely natural ingredients. Rather than synthetic these are unaltered natural extracts, where the chemistry is kept as close to nature as possible. While true whole foods are best, the majority of nutritional supplements are synthetic or semi-synthetic. All aforementioned formulas are truly 100% natural, completely unaltered. All these products are fully wild. In this regard many of the substances are handpicked and minimally processed. That is what makes the products of North American Herb & Spice Co. unique. This is also why by taking the North American formulas the need for other supplements, such as synthetic multiple vitamins, minerals, and highly processed herbs, is greatly reduced, even eliminated. The fact is this is all the individual needs. Once the virus is purged, the cancer will be destroyed. This is the cause-and-effect approach which makes these products unique.

It was Max Gerson, M.D., who demonstrated the potential toxicity of synthetic supplements. As demonstrated by his research the regular intake of such vitamins, which are made from coal tar, increases tumor growth. This is why only natural-source supplements must be consumed. It is North American Herb & Spice which specializes in such natural-source formulas. The wild spice extracts, the crude pumpkinseed oil (that is the Pumpkinol), the fortified royal jelly (that is the Royal Power), the crude red sour grape powder, the wild greens, Oil of Black Seed, and the cranberry extract: all are true whole food supplements. All such substances are antiviral agents but are also foods with cleansing powers. Thus, they are safe in large amounts for any age or circumstance.

Protocol for the purging of SV40 and other stealth viruses

This protocol is based upon years of experience in the treatment of chronic viral infections as well as vaccine injury. The spice oils, derived from wild growing plants, have been shown to purge from cells a wide range of viruses. These are the most powerful antiviral substances known. Also, various plant flavonoids are antiviral. Some of the most potent plant flavonoids known are included in this purge.

- Oil of wild oregano (P73)—two droppersful twice daily. For tough cases use the SuperStrength version of Oreganol P73 at the same dosage.
- OregaBiotic multiple spice capsules—two to three capsules twice daily. For difficult conditions increase dose to three

capsules three times daily. The OregaBiotic should be taken with food or juice. (OregaRESP is also effective in purging the virus)

- Oreganol Juice of wild Oregano—one ounce twice daily.
- Garlex cold-pressed garlic oil—two droppersful twice daily.
- Oil of Black Seed—one tablespoon daily.
- Neuroloft essence or capsules—if using the capsules, two twice daily, and if using the essence, one ounce twice daily.
- Purely-C a (natural vitamin C complex)—two or three capsules twice daily.
- GrapeFast (wild grape cleansing substance)—take forty drops twice daily (resveratrol is highly antiviral)

Note: Remain on the antiviral purge for at least 90 days or, preferably, six months. For difficult cases it may be necessary to continue this for up to a year. The viruses are deeply entrenched. It takes a major effort to purge them.

Optional

- EFA Orega (essential fatty acids for acting as a barrier against cancer)—forty drops twice daily.
- CranFlush (to flush out noxious germs through the kidneys; wild cranberry extract is a potent germicide)—one dropperful twice daily.
- Inflam-eez natural antiinflammatory enzymes—two or more capsules twice daily on an empty stomach.
- LivaClenz (for purging hidden viruses from the liver)— take three capsules twice daily with food.
- Thyroset (for balancing thyroid function, greatly aids the immune system)—three capsules twice daily.
- Royal Power (for balancing the adrenal glands and immune system)—three capsules once or twice daily; the ideal time to take this is in the morning.

Treatment protocol for children

- Oil of wild oregano (use only the edible type, P73)—two or more drops under the tongue or in juice/honey twice daily.
- Kid-e-Kare wild spice oil gelcaps—one or two capsules twice daily.
- Kid-e-Kare throat spray (wild bush cherry-based plus essential oils)—spray as often as possible in the back of the throat.
- Kid-e-Kare massage oil with antiseptic essential oils—rub up and down the spine as much as possible once or twice daily; also rub on the feet.
- OregaMax capsules—maximum strength wild herb, take two capsules twice daily. These are large capsules, so it may be necessary to open them and add to food or beverages. The wild herb is a rich source of flavonoids and trace minerals. It is a natural mineral supplement, rich in calcium, magnesium, phosphorus, and zinc.
- Oreganol Juice of wild Oregano—one or two tablespoons daily in juice/water.
- EFA Orega—twenty drops twice daily.

Note: When taking high doses of spice oils, as above, it is necessary to replenish the healthy bacteria, which may be to a degree killed. To do so use the European strains of Lactobacillus acidophilus and bifidus, that is the Health-Bac, a half teaspoon or more at night in a small amount of warm water. Ideally, take right before bedtime. This is a purely vegetable origin healthy bacterial supplement. It is free of any pork or human derivatives.

General liver cleanse for boosting the regenerative capacity

This is to ease the pressure on the immune system, particularly during the SV40 purge. This will greatly aid the overall effort. In other words, by consistently cleansing the liver of toxins there is an increased capacity to clear vaccine viruses from the tissues. What's more, the liver cleanse itself helps purge viruses. This cleanse should always be performed simultaneously with the SV40 cleanse.

- LivaClenz—two or three capsules with every meal or for people with low body weight, two with every meal. Ideally, take with a fat-containing meal.
- GreensFlush—two or more droppersful twice daily under the tongue. This is an aid to obstructed bowels and/or constipation. The Flush is ideal for maintaining normal function in the colon. This greatly aids the healing effort.
- GrapeFast—three or more droppersful twice daily. The wild berry flavonoids are cleansing, primarily for the blood and colon: they are also antiviral.
- Health-Bac (to repopulate the colon and take the stress off the liver)—take 1/2 to one teaspoon in warm water twice daily.

Note: Children can also follow our liver-cleansing plan.

Note: MSG may also be listed on labels as hydrolyzed vegetable protein, which is about 40% MSG by weight, or even natural flavors.

Appendix B

RELIGIOUS EXEMPTION FROM VACCINATION

DATE _____

I _____, parent of _____,

claim religious exemption under section 167.181 RSMo due to religious and moral convictions. My objections are listed below as follows:

Public Law 97-280, passed by the 97th Congress of the United States of America, declares the Bible to be the "Word of God" and directs citizens to "study and apply the teachings of the Holy Scriptures. The Bible teaches that the truthfulness of an issue is to be sought and should stand on no less than two or more witnesses." (Deuteronomy 19:15)

A diligent search for truth on the safety and effectiveness of vaccinations reveals there are many studied, informed and qualified witnesses who have found and teach that there are serious health risks involved with vaccinations. Even Senate Bill 732 before the 103rd Congress of the United States known as the "Comprehensive Child Health Immunization Act of 1993" made known the fact that there are risks to vaccines. The following words are from that bill: "Vaccine information materials should be simplified to ensure that parents can understand the *benefits and risks* of vaccines" (emphasis added).

The Bible teaches that there are clean and unclean animals and that God's people are not to put the unclean into their bodies (Deuteronomy 14). Furthermore, the Bible teaches that "Ye shall not eat of anything that dieth of itself" (Deuteronomy 14:21) and "that flesh with the life thereof, which is the blood thereof, shall ye not eat." (Genesis 9:4) Vaccines are often made of, or embody, fetuses or eggs of said unclean creatures. The process of creating the vaccine often causes said creatures to die in the process (that is, dieth of itself). Many vaccines are made in or of the blood of diseased animals.

"What know ye not that your body is the temple of the Holy Ghost which is in you, which ye have of God, and ye are not your own. For ye are bought with a price: therefore glorify God in your body, and in your spirit, which are God's." (I Corinthians 6:19, 20)

The Bible teaches that we are not to harm or wrong our neighbor. (Romans 13:10: James 2:8) Our decision to decline vaccinations does not wrong or threaten our neighbor. If vaccinations are truly effective, then vaccinated neighbors would be in no danger from someone who is not vaccinated. Also, statistics show that those NOT vaccinated are less likely to expose their neighbor to harmful pathogens (that are contained in the vaccinations).

Hepatitis B Not Highly Contagious—unlike other infectious diseases for which vaccines have been developed and mandated in the U.S., hepatitis B is not common in childhood and is not highly contagious. Hepatitis B is primarily an adult disease transmitted through infected body fluids, most frequently infected blood, and is prevalent in high risk populations such as needle-using drug addicts, sexually promiscuous heterosexual and homosexual adults, residents and staff of custodial institutions such as prisons, health care workers exposed to blood, persons who require repeated blood transfusions and babies born to infected mothers.

According to *CDC Prevention Guidelines: A Guide to Action* (1997), a book written by federal public health officials at the U.S. government Centers for Disease Control (CDC), "the sources of [hepatitis B] infection for most cases include intravenous drug use (28%) heterosexual contact with infected persons or multiple partners (22%) and homosexual activity (9%)." According to *Harrison's Principles of Internal Medicine* (1944), mother-to-child transmission of hepatitis B "is common in North America and western Europe.

Although CDC officials have made statements that hepatitis B is easy to catch through sharing toothbrushes or razors, Eric Mast, M.D., Chief of the Surveillance Section, Hepatitis Branch of the CDC, stated in a 1997 public hearing that: "although [the hepatitis B virus] is present in moderate concentrations in saliva, it's not transmitted commonly by casual contact."

Some of the ingredients of our current vaccines are:
(1) **formaldehyde**, used in production of resins, plastics, and foam insulation, and as a preservative, disinfectant, and antibacterial food additive. It is a known carcinogen (can initiate a new cancer), commonly used to embalm corpses.

(2) **Thimerosal**, a mercury derivative. The heavy metal mercury is toxic to the central nervous system and not easily eliminated from the body. "Aluminum, formaldehyde and mercury"—including the mercury in "silver" dental fillings and amalgams (see Chapter 9)—"have a long history of documented hazardous effects including cancer, neurological damage" such as multiple sclerosis, Lou Gehrig's disease, "and death."

Studies report, "Thimerosal inhibits phagocytes, one of the body's most vital immune defenses in blood." Then what effect will it have on healthy human cells after it is injected into the bloodstream? Jamie Murphy, a concerned nonprofessional observer, asks, "Who would take chemicals that are carcinogenic in rats, are used in the manufacture of inks, dyes, explosives, wrinkle-proof fabrics, home insulation, and embalming fluid—and inject them into the delicate body of a baby?"

Among other vaccine ingredients are **aluminum phosphate**, **aluminum adjuvants, alum, and acetone**; **phenol** is included in allergy injections. "Benzoic acid, a preservative whose injection into rats causes tremors, convulsions, and death, is added. And then vaccine makers add decomposing animal proteins, such as pig or horse blood, cow pox pus, rabbit brain tissue, duck egg protein, and dog kidney tissue."

A glance at further steps in vaccine making is no less disturbing. To produce a "live" virus vaccine, such as MMR (measles/mumps/rubella), the virus is passed through animal tissue several times to reduce its potency. **Measles virus is passed through chick embryos, polio virus through monkey kidney, and the rubella virus is passed through the dissected organs of an aborted human fetus.**

"Killed' vaccines are 'inactivated' through heat, radiation, or chemicals. The weakened germ is then strengthened with antibody boosters and stabilizers. This is done by the addition of **drugs, antibiotics** and **toxic disinfectants:** neomycin, streptomycin, sodium chloride, sodium hydroxide, aluminum hydroxide, aluminum hydrochloride, sorbitol, hydrolyzed gelatin, formaldehyde [again], and thimerosal [again]."

Injected straight into the child's bloodstream—bypassing the cellular immune system, one-half of our protective immunity mechanism—those materials destroy stores of protective nutrients in the tiny body. So it is not hard to see why epidemic vaccines worsen health throughout life.

Only two single-antigen pediatric hepatitis B vaccines exist on the US market, Engerix-B (SmithKline Beecham) and Recombivax HB (Merck). Both contain thimerosal and 12.5 micrograms of mercury per 0.5 ml dose.

Bibliography

Adams, J. H. 1967. *Viruses and Colds: The Modern Plague.* New York: American Elsevier Publ. Co.

Barbanti-Brodano, G., et al. 2004. Simian virus 40 infection in humans and association with human diseases: results and hypotheses. *Virology.* 318:1-9.

Bayly, M. B. 1956. *The Story of the Salk Anti-Poliomyelitis Vaccine.* (as found on the Web site, Whale, supplied by J. Wantling.)

Berg, R. H. 1946. *The Challenge of Polio.* New York: The Dial Press.

Bergsagel, D. J., et al. 1992. DNA sequences similar to those of simian virus 40 in ependymomas and choroid plexus tumors of childhood. *New England Journal of Medicine.* 326:988-993.

Bolognesi, D. P. 1976. Potential leukemia virus subunit vaccines: discussion. *Can. Res.* 36(2, pt. 2): 655-56.

Bravo, M. P., et al. 1988. Association between the occurrence of antibodies to simian vaculoating virus 40 and bladder cancer in male smokers. *Neoplasia.* 35:285-288.

Butel, J. S., et al. 2003. Association between SV40 and non-Hodgkin's lymphoma. *Leuk Lymphoma.* 3:S33-9.

Butel, J. S., Jafar, S., Stewart, A. R., and J. A. Lednicky. 1998. Detection of authentic SV40 DNA sequences in human brain and bone tumors. *Dev. Biol. Stand.* 94:23-32.

Butel, J. S. and J. A. Lednicky. 1999. Cell and molecular biology of simian virus 40: implications for human infections and disease. *J. Natl Cancer Inst.* 91:119-134.

Carbone, M., et al. 1996. SV-40 like sequences in human bone tumors. Oncogene. 13:527-535.

Colon, V. F., et al. 1968. Vaccinia necrosum as a clue to lymphatic lymphoma. *Geriatrics.* 23:81-82.

Cournoyer, C. 1995. *What About Immunizations? Exposing the Vaccine Philosophy.* Santa Cruz: Nelson's Books.

Davies, D. H. 1999. *Infection and Immunity.* London: Taylor & Francis.

Deichmann, W. B. and H. W. Gerarde. 1969. *Toxicology of Drugs and Chemicals.* New York: Academic Press.

Dolcetti, R., et al. 2003. Simian virus 40 sequences in human lymphoblastoid B-cell lines. *J. Virol.* 77:1595.

Geissler, E. 1986. SV40 in human intracranial tumors: passenger virus or oncogenic "hit-and-run agent?" *Z. Klin. Med.* 41:493.

Geissler, E. 1990. SV40 and human brain tumors. Progress in *Medical Virology.* 37:211-222.

Glathe, H., et al. 1977. Evidence of tumorigenic activity of candidate cell substrate in vaccine production by the use of anti-lymphocyte serum. *Devel. Biol. Std.* 34:145.

Hornig, M., Chian, D. and W. I. Lipkin. 2004. Neurotoxic effects of postnatal thimerasol are mouse strain dependent. *Molecular Psychiatry*, pp. 1-13.

Hugoson, G., et al. 1968. The occurrence of bovine leukosis following the introduction of babesiosis vaccination. *Bilb. Haemat.* 30:157.

Hultman, P. and H. Hansson-Georgiadis. 1999. Methyl mercury-induced autoimmunity in mice. *Toxicol. Appl Pharmacol.* 154:203-211.

Ingram, Cass (Kaasem). 2003. *Nutrition Tests for Better Health.* Buffalo Grove, IL: Knowledge House.

Ingram, Cass (Kaasem). 2003. *Natural Cures for Killer Germs.* Buffalo Grove, IL: Knowledge House.

Innis, M. D. 1968. Oncogenesis and poliomyelitis vaccine. *Nature.* 219:972-73.

Krieg, P., et al. Episomal simian virus 40 genomes in human brain tumors. *Proc. Nat. Acad. Sci.* 78:6446-50.

Kumagai, T., Nagai, K., Okui, T., et al. 2004. Poor immune responses to influenza vacinnation in infants. *Pediatric Allegy and Infectious Diseases Society* (Sapporo, Kumagai Ped. Clin.).

Lednicky, J. A., et al. 1995. Natural simian virus 40 strains are present in human choroid plexus and ependymoma tumors. *Virology.* 212:710-717.

Lednicky, J. A., Stewart, A. R., Jenkins, J. J. 3rd, Finegold, M. J. and Butel, J. S. 1997. SV40 DNA in human osteosarcomas show sequence variation among T-antigen genes. *In. J. Cancer.* 4:791.

Maas, K., et al. 2002. Cutting edge: molecular portrait of human autoimmune disease. *J. Immunol.* 169:5-9.

McBean, E. 1993. *The Poisoned Needle.* Mokelumne Hill: Health Research.

Miller, N. Z. 1996. *Immunizations: The People Speak!* Santa Fe: New Atlantean Press.

Miller, N. Z. 1996. *Immunization: Theory vs Realty.* Sante Fe: New Atlantean Press.

Meinke, W., et al. 1979. Simian virus 40-related DNA sequences in a human brain tumor. *Neurology.* 29:1590-1594.

Martini, M., et al. 1995. Human brain tumors and simian virus 40. *J. Nat. Can. Inst.* 87:1331.

Martini, M., et al. 1996. SV-40 early region and large T antigen in human brain tumors, peripheral blood cells, and sperm fluids from healthy individuals. *Cancer Research.* 56:4820-4825.

Nielson. J. B. and P. Hultman. 2002. Mercury-induced autoimmunity in mice. *Environ. Health Perspect.* 110 (Suppl. 5):877.

Howe, H. A. 1942. *Neural Mechanisms in Poliomyelitis.* New York: The Commonwealth Fund.

Omokoku, B. and S. Castells. 1981. Post-DPT inoculation cervical lymphadenitis in children. *N. Y. State J. Med.* Oct, 81(11): 1667-1668.

Pass, H. I. Kennedy, R. C., and M. Carbone. 1966. Evidence for and implications of SV-40-like sequences in human mesotheliomas. *Important Advances in Oncology,* pp. 89-108.

Pichichero, M. E., et al. 2002. Mercury concentrations and metabolism in infants receiving vaccines containing thimerasol: a descriptive study. *Lancet.* 360:1737-1741.

Poliomyelitis. 1949. Papers and Discussons Presented at the First Internationial Poliomyelitis Conference. International Poliomyelitis Congress. Philadelphia: J. B. Lippincott.

Poliomyelitis. 1960. Papers and Discussions Presented at the *Fifth International Poliomyelitis Conference,* Copenhagen, Denmark, July 26-28. Philadelphia: J. B. Lippincott Co.

Rock, A. 1996. The Lethal Dangers of the Billion Dollar Vaccine Business. *Money.* Dec., pp. 161.

Rosa, F. W., et al. 1988. Absence of antibody response to simian virus 40 after inoculation with killed-poliovirus vaccine of mother's offspring with neurological tumors. *New England Journal of Medicine.* 318:1469.

Rosa, F. W., et al. 1988. Response to neurological tumors in offspring after inoculation of mothers with killed poliovirus vaccine. *New England Journal of Medicine.* 319:1226.

Schaeffer, M. and R. S. Muckenfuss. *Experimental Poliomyelitis.* The National Foundation for Infantile Paralysis.

Scherneck, S., et al. 1979. Isolation of an SV-40-like papovavirus from a human glioblastoma. *In. J. Cancer.* 24:523.

Shah, K. and N. Nathanson. 1976. Human exposure to SV40. *American Journal of Epidemiology.* 103:1-12.

Sheibner, V. 1993. *Vaccination: the Medical Assault on the Immune System.* Australian Print Group.

Shivapurkar, N., et al. 1961. Presence of simian virus 40 DNA sequences in human lymphoid and hematopoietic malignancies and their relationships to aberrant promoter methylation of multiple genes. *JAMA*. 178:1125-1127. *Cancer Res.* 1:64.

Snider, A. 1963. Near Disaster with the Salk Vaccine. *Science Digest*. (Dec.)

Soriano, F., et al. 1974. Simian virus 40 in a human cancer. *Nature*. 249:421.

Stoian, M., et al. 1987. Possible relation between viruses and oromaxillofacial tumors. II. Research on the presence of SV40 antigen and specific antibodies in patients with oromaxillofacial tumors. *Virologie*. 38:35-40.

Stoian, M., et al. 1987. Possible relation between viruses and oromaxillofacial tumors. II. Detection of SV40 antigen and of antiSV40 antibodies in patients with parotid gland tumors. *Virologie*. 38:41-46.

Tabuchi, K. 1978. Screening of human brain tumors for SV-40-related T-antigen. *International Journal of Cancer*. 21:12-17.

Thomas, S. 1927. Tetanus vaccination. *J. Inf. Dis.*, Nov.

Uhlmann, V., et al. 2002. Potential viral pathogenic mechanism for new variant inflammatory bowel disease. *Mol. Pathol.* 55:84.

Vilchez, R. A. and J. S. Butel. 2003. SV40 in human cancers and non-Hodgkin's lymphoma. *Ocongene*. 22:5164-72.

Vilchez, R. A. and J. S. Butel. 2003. Simian virus 40 and its association with human lymphomas. *Curr. Oncol. Rep.* 5:372.

Vilchez, R. A., et al. 2003. Simian virus 40 in human cancers. *Am. J. Med.* 114:675.

Vojdani, A., et al. 2003. Infections, toxic chemicals and dietary peptides binding to lymphocyte receptors and tissue enzymes are major instigators of autoimmunity in autism. *In. J. Immunopathol. Pharmacol.* 16: 189-199.

C. Frh. von Pirquet, and Bela Schick, 1951. *Serum Sickness*. Baltimore: Williams & Wilkins Co.

Wallace, A. R. 1898. *Vaccination a Delusion - Its Penal Enforcement a Crime*. London.

Weiss, A. F., et al. 1975. Simian virus 40-related antigens in three human meningiomas with defined chromosomal loss. *Proc. Natl. Acad. Sci.* 72(2):609.

Westphal, G. A., et al. 2000. Homozygous gene deletions of the gluthathione-S-transferases M1 and T are associated with thimerasol sensitization. *In. Arch. Occup. Environ. Health*. 73:384-388.

Whitelock, O. V., Furness, F. N., Collins, B., and E. W. White. 1960. Care and Diseases of the Research Monkey. *Annals of the New York Academy of Sciences* (85):735-992. New York: The Academy.

Index

A

Addison's disease, 55, 85, 183, 246, 270
Afghanistan, 230
Africa, 8, 32, 86, 275, 293
AIDS, 34, 55, 56, 259, 300
Albumin, 57, 179, 240, 269
  in urine, 269
ALS, 65, 94, 115, 137, 153, 181, 182, 183, 255, 257, 301, 309, 316
Alzheimer's Disease, 17, 85, 153, 179-183, 223, 225, 257, 269, 309
Amalgam fillings, 139, 141, 149
American Cancer Society, 7, 206
American Cyanamid, 169, 177, 178, 194
Amino acids, 106, 318, 319
Ankylosing spondylitis, 29, 48, 56, 85, 113, 207, 268, 300, 301
Antibiotics, 42, 89, 107, 109, 110, 123, 254, 281
Antibody-antigen complexes, 240
Arney, 131, 132
Arnow, L. E., 228
Arthritis, 29, 47, 55, 56, 96, 113, 179, 182, 183, 184, 207, 246, 268, 269, 277, 293, 295, 297, 300, 301
Asthma, 47, 95, 101, 186, 192, 244, 246, 293, 295, 309

Attention deficit, 17, 29, 85, 135, 179, 207, 231, 256, 268, 269, 277, 301, 309
Autism, 17, 29, 85, 115, 130, 133, 134, 135, 179, 190, 207, 222, 231, 256, 269, 277, 301, 304, 309
Autoimmune disorders, 81, 95, 98, 182, 183, 186, 207, 246, 257, 288, 309
Aventis Pasteur, 122, 126, 231, 232
A-Panama, 126
A-New Caledonia, 126

B

Bacillus subtilus, 76
Barnes, Ida, M.D., 35
Baskin, Dr. David, 115
Bastian, Frank O., M.D., 106
Bayly, M. B., 63, 119, 154, 160
Bell, Robert, M.D., 278
Bell's palsy, 80, 180-183, 231, 255, 269
Benjamin, Mark, 224
Berg, Roland H., 208, 209
Bible, 84
Bile, 311, 317, 318
Bison, 319, 322
Bloch, Scott J., 114, 115
Bodian, David, 165, 167, 169
Bone marrow, 48, 78, 79, 89, 94, 104, 244, 245, 321
Breast-feeding, 190, 226
British Medical Journal, 284, 285, 293, 296
British Ministry of Health, 68
Bronchitis, 186, 246, 269, 301
Butel, 283
B-Shangdong, 126

336